I Just Want to Function!

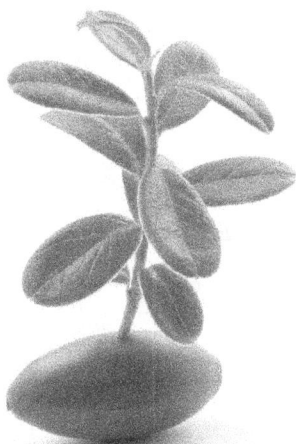

I Just Want to Function!

FUNCTIONAL MEDICINE:
THE BASICS OF FEELING BETTER

"My mission is to reach as many people as possible with the goal of giving them the basic knowledge of functional medicine, what it is, and how it can help with chronic conditions like fibromyalgia, chronic fatigue syndrome, anxiety, depression, and a host of other chronic health conditions."

Cindy Cotsiopoulos, RN

I Just Want to Function!
Functional Medicine: The Basics of Feeling Better

For information about this title or to order other books and/or electronic media, contact the publisher:

Your Functional Health Basics LLC
www.functionalhealthbasics.com
Cindy@functionalhealthbasics.com

ISBNs:
979-8-9862161-0-2 (softcover)
979-8-9862161-1-9 (eBook)

Printed in the United States of America

Cover and Interior design: 1106 Design

To my husband John, the hardest working man I know. Above all, thank you for your love and loyalty, and for allowing me to use my time and our resources to find the answers and to do what I needed to do to improve my health. Physically and financially, repeatedly, you made up for my lack when I didn't have the ability, at times, to work as a nurse while at the same time being a good wife and mom. I love you!

CONTENTS

CONTENTS

CONTENTS

PREFACE

It was 2015 and physically I had felt worse than I had ever felt in my life! And that is saying something, because for the previous three decades I had already been struggling with chronic health problems that left me dragging and in pain all the time. Mid-nineties, when I was in my late twenties, I started having chronic health problems and was first diagnosed with hypothyroidism and then fibromyalgia. Since then it's been one diagnosis after another. My son has had many chronic health issues as well. It was only after learning about functional medicine in 2015 that I started getting to the root of my health problems as well as my son's. Today, in my mid-fifties, I feel better than I did in my twenties, thirties, and forties.

Since 2015, I have found my new passion in learning all that I can about functional medicine and figuring out how I can help others. Functional medicine is based on scientifically finding the root cause of chronic illness. With the improvement of my own health, friends and family have taken notice and often ask me for advice on how to feel better, lose weight, and other ways to improve their own well-being. Depending on their question, the answer can occasionally be very simple and straightforward, but more often than not it's complex. That's why I've written this book; I want to educate on the deeper things that a fifteen-minute conversation with someone wouldn't even begin to touch on.

I received my nursing education in the late eighties and early nineties and became a licensed practical nurse in 1987 and then a registered nurse in 1990. Through those years I worked mostly with special needs children in home settings. Because of the health of my son and mother, in addition to my own, I wasn't able to be a "career" nurse. There were many years I didn't even work at all. During a health crisis in 2015, I came across Dr. Hyman's *The Blood Sugar Solution 10-Day Detox Diet Cookbook*. It taught me about functional medicine, which led to a more in-depth elimination diet overseen by Alissa Segersten and Tom Malterre, MS, CN, authors of *The Whole Life Nutrition Cookbook*, *Nourishing Meals*, and *The Elimination Diet*. This was the turning point in my health. As my health was improving, I wanted to shout out to the world about how functional medicine helped me get my life back. In 2017, I developed a website that was mainly for educational purposes. But I wasn't really sure how I was going to go about my mission to help others.

A lot happened in my life from 2017 to 2019 where I wasn't able to do more than my website for helping others. Early in 2020, I was entering a field altogether different from healthcare because I really didn't want to return to nursing. It's not that I didn't love helping people; it was just that taking care of sick children was emotionally taxing. Driven by my crazy passion for organizing, I was just getting my business of being an organizer up and running and had two clients when the COVID-19 Pandemic hit. I could see at this point that home organizing wasn't going to work out as a source of income for the time being. So I fearfully went back into nursing, taking care of medically fragile children as a financial necessity. Turns out that my fears were not justified. I have been blessed to work with a wonderful child and her family.

My passion to get the word out about functional medicine still hadn't left me, however. During this time I came across a course that taught me how to become a certified functional health coach, and the idea that I could actually help others in the field of functional medicine started to become real to me. So I started planning my business of taking on clients as a certified functional health coach. As I did that, I tried to figure out how I could help others in a way that would be low stress for them, not overwhelming, and yet give them the ability to become autonomous in their own growth.

You know the saying, "If you give a man a fish, you feed him for a day. If you teach a man to fish, you feed him for a lifetime." The same is true with health and wellness. If people can be taught where to "fish" for answers, they can be empowered to take control of their own health and wellness, and then they can navigate their own health journey. So I decided to put together my knowledge of functional medicine and my organizing skills to formulate this educational guide and workbook so I can help you with your wellness journey.

ACKNOWLEDGMENTS

First, I want to thank all the thousands of medical professionals who have had the courage to talk about the root cause as a solution to the rise of many autoimmune illnesses and other chronic ailments, rather than the many bandages that abound in modern medicine. Your own stories of recovery from poor health, and your abundant knowledge has inspired me to pull together the basics in a simple way to reach and inspire others to take their first steps on their journey to better health.

A special thanks specifically to those whom I have learned from: **Dr. Joel Fuhrman, M.D**. In your book *Eat to Live* and that wonderful San Diego Seminar in 2013, you gave me that start on the right path to understanding nutrition, and the role it plays in our health and vitality. **Dr. Mark Hyman M.D.:** the word "functional Medicine," and the meaning behind it, came into my life through your books at a critical time in my life. You started me on the path for discovering my own root causes to my own autoimmune struggles. Through you I found out about The Elimination Diet program by **Allissa Segersten** and **Tom Malterre MS, CN.** Allissa Segersten, thank you for your amazing recipes that fill the needs of many, no matter what their dietary needs are. Your website and books have all been amazing! I'm looking forward to finding more amazing recipes on your new platform Nourishing Meals. I've even put a link to it on my own website because it is a valuable tool for anyone learning to navigate new dietary options. **Izabella Wentz PharmD, FASCFASCP:** thank you for The Thyroid Secret Summit and your book *Hashimoto's Protocol.* I have learned so much from you about the thyroid. Putting your own Hashimoto's into remission has been an inspiration for me as I have successfully gotten my own autoimmune levels to normal. My doctor, **Dr. Yvonne Karney M.D.** for helping me to navigate my own health journey and finding those answers that I couldn't discover on my own and for teaching me even more about functional medicine than what I have read about. **Chris Kresser M.S., L.Ac.:** for your wonderful ongoing education that continues to keep me learning, growing, and sharing with others. All of these professionals continue to influence my knowledge and growth way beyond this book.

Writing a book is one thing, but knowing what to do with it after it was written was another. A big thank you to author and writing coach **Sara Connell**. Your workshops just seem to come at the right times when I was left wondering what to do with my manuscript. Thank you to the team at **1106 Design** who helped me to polish my manuscript into a work of art and professionalism. **Michele DeFilippo,** you have a great group of people working for you. **Ronda** and **Doran** have been easy to work with as well as all the others that I haven't had the pleasure to know by name.

Thank you to my dear friends who read my manuscript for this book or the workbook and gave me feedback. I really appreciate that you took the time from your busy schedules to help me out. **Collene**, thank you for reading my manuscript and letting me know that you felt that I was talking about your own struggles in my book. It gave me the hope that anyone who has suffered with chronic illness will come away feeling that they can relate and that there are solutions. **Dee** and **Joan**, thank you for using your teacher and editor skills with my workbook. I'm blessed to have such great loyal friends who have been willing to help me out. I'll get those cookies to you Joan! Haha!

Finally, to those most important to me. A special thanks, with deep love and appreciation, to those dearest to my heart. My loyal, hardworking husband **John** and loving son **Austin** who have lovingly given me space at home to write this book and workbook. Thank you for your love and encouragement. My dearest loving daughter **Ashley** and my awesome, devoted son-in-law **Evan** who have also supported me and encouraged me. Thank you both for also taking the time to read my book and workbook and then giving me the feedback that I needed. Yes, I needed to hear that the non-medical population would have no idea what I was talking about when I used medical terms. (I let the editor find those for me. Thanks Doran! Ha-ha!) I love all four of you and am a very blessed wife and mom.

INTRODUCTION

"What is going on here? Why am I sleeping all the time? How can I be a good mom if I can't get off the couch or out of bed? How can I fulfill the obligations I have for my family and my spiritual volunteer commitments?"

These are the questions that I was asking myself in 2015. I was dragging myself through life, and this wasn't the first time, but this time it was worse. I was plagued with chronic pain in my neck, back, shoulders, and hips. I was not sleeping well at night. I couldn't get off the couch during the day. At times, I was gasping for air. I was struggling to breathe! It was as if, at moments, my lungs had a mind of their own and were forgetting to breathe. In my mind, I was saying, "What if I stop breathing in my sleep?" and "Is this how I want to go out?"

From the time I was little to my early twenties, I had chronic ear and sinus infections, leading to constant antibiotic use. I also had a positive TB skin reaction from working in healthcare, requiring nine months of prophylactic antibiotics. Only later did I learn about how antibiotics mess with the gut and lead to other chronic health conditions.

In my late twenties came the real chronic health struggles that altered the quality of my life. I had two miscarriages, and with the two babies I successfully carried, I failed to go into labor and provide enough milk. "Why couldn't I have normal pregnancies like everyone else?" I kept asking myself. I developed an oral allergy syndrome to raw nectarines, apples, and cherries. In addition to seasonal and environmental allergies, in my mid-twenties I became sensitive to various everyday environmental chemicals. I developed allergy-induced asthma, headaches, and brain fog. I had chronic symptoms of fatigue, bloating, GI gas, chronic widespread pain, ringing in my ears, exercise intolerance, poor memory, and anxiety. The list goes on and on. Through those years, the answers started to come, little by little. I was given diagnoses like hypothyroidism (later correctly diagnosed as Hashimoto's thyroiditis), fibromyalgia, postpartum depression, seasonal depression, celiac disease, Lyme disease, and Epstein-Barr virus (EBV).

So why was I sicker in 2016 than in the previous years? Beginning in 2014, my family was displaced for eight months because the sale of our home was unexpectedly quick. We lived with family for much of the time, and when we finally found a home, we did some work on it before moving in. Within a month of moving in, my health was worse than ever because of a combination of excessive stress, poor eating while on the run, mold exposure, and a higher level of chemical exposure than I was used to. My bucket of tolerance was overflowing at a critical level.

This was when functional medicine came into my life. Functional medicine scientifically gets to the root cause of illness based on how our body was designed to function. In the first chapter of this book, I dive deeper into what functional medicine is and the process it takes to get to the answers. I finally had the information that empowered me to gain control of my health and enjoy life fully because I could actually function. I began to see that my issues were more than just food sensitivities. So in 2017, I consulted a functional medicine practitioner, an MD, who specializes in finding the root cause of various health issues. Some major root causes for my health issues were environmental toxins, food sensitivities, SAD (Standard American Diet), SIBO (small intestinal bacterial overgrowth), nutrient deficiencies such as vitamin D and B12, a copper/zinc imbalance, leaky gut, and adrenal issues related to major stresses and managing those stresses poorly. By changing my diet to eliminate processed foods and foods known to be inflammatory, addressing nutrient deficiencies, removing any toxins in my environment, and focusing on the way I manage stress (still working on that one), I have been able to greatly improve my ability to function and be healthy. The process of feeling better has been like peeling away the layers of an onion. Layer by layer, I am able to function better.

I can now go through the day without having to take a nap. I sleep pretty well. And most exciting is my ability to run with my dog and not experience any pain. We are not talking about marathons here, just sprinting at the park—ha-ha! But at fifty-five I can do it again and without pain. I've also had a dramatic reduction in gut issues and an unintended but very welcome weight loss of thirty pounds all within six months back in 2017 and 2018. By the end of 2021, I have reached fifty pounds down and feel better at fifty-five than I did in my twenties. I still have challenges that I need to address but sticking with the mentality of this being a *journey* instead of finding a quick fix has been the key for me to overcome health obstacles and optimize my ability to live and function successfully.

As for my son? When my son was born in 1999, because of my low milk supply, we supplemented and discovered that he had a dairy allergy. Other multiple food and environmental allergies and sensitivities were diagnosed. He has had chronic ear and sinus infections, asthma, abdominal pain, chronic nausea and vomiting, ADHD, GERD (gastroesophageal reflux disease), anxiety, and depression.

Just before he turned three he began having seizures and at one point an EEG showed that he was having up to two hundred episodes of seizure activity *per day*! Thankfully, within a year, we finally had them under control with conventional medicine.

In 2017, he was diagnosed with chronic Lyme disease, and we tried the functional medicine approach with him. At that time he was seventeen, so he was on a different self-destructive mission. Unfortunately (or fortunately, depending on how you look at it), in 2018, he was in a severe automobile accident that has compounded the struggles he faces. But it was the wake-up call that got him to take a good hard look at his life. He has been moving gradually forward and conquering his challenges one at a time, and in 2020 he was diagnosed with celiac disease by my functional medicine MD. As of 2021, he went gluten free and is now off medication for GERD and has seen many other health improvements through addressing the root causes of his health challenges. At the beginning of 2022, he approached me and told me that he is ready to go further on his journey. He's sick and tired of his physical and emotional struggles and is ready to change his diet further and do whatever work he has to do so he can function his best. He is tired of suffering! He has started neuro rehabilitation treatment for the brain injury from his accident and is now seeing a functional medicine practitioner to address the chronic health issues he deals with daily.

And that's how it really goes for all of us. It's a *journey* that we must individually be willing to take in order to succeed. We take the first step by educating ourselves and then, depending on who we are and our budget, we start to take baby steps, gigantic steps, or somewhere-in-between steps. Some of us reach the end of our rope, others run out of options, and for many of us, it's life or death. Where are you on your journey?

WHAT WILL YOU LEARN
IN THIS BOOK?

Have you ever bought a book on health and wellness hoping to get straight to the answers? Then this book is for you. I've designed it to be an easy-to-understand approach to help those seeking answers. It contains basic information for those who may feel overwhelmed with too much information. And for those who want to learn and understand more, I have provided references to reliable websites and books.

In the first section of this book, you will find seven pillars of health and wellness. I break these pillars down so that you can discover areas you may want to explore more in your own health journey. You can read them all or pick the ones you feel are beneficial to your own journey.

In the second section, I talk about supplements. For instance, just the other day my daughter called me from the store looking for specific supplements for her husband. She was standing in the supplement aisle overwhelmed with the choices. Perhaps you have been in the same position, standing there in the aisle faced with thirty different vitamin-C brands and types, all claiming to be the best. You start to feel a heavy weight over your chest. Perhaps your palms start to perspire. At the very least, you feel a mild ache in your temples or along the back of your neck. Stress, tension—it can be overwhelming for many. So I talk a little about certain supplements and what you want to look for and what you want to avoid. I also mention cautions to consider when taking them and what to look for in a good quality supplement.

In the third section, I talk about specific health areas you may be interested in. These are common conditions or symptoms individuals may be dealing with and the functional medicine verses the conventional approach to managing them. In the end, we are all individuals who will make different decisions. So I hope the information you gather will help you in making the most informed decision for your unique circumstances.

WHY THIS APPROACH?

What is unique about the approach of this book and accompanying downloadable workbook is that you can pick where you want to start and decide how much you can take on. Pick the pillar of health that is least stressful to you or the one you most identify with your goals. Each person is different. Maybe you just have one problem to address, like lack of sleep for instance. Then that will be all you need. Pick two or more if you are very motivated or have more challenges. Start there by learning and then applying what you can in a progressive way.

It takes time to work through these pillars if you are hardly functioning. It took me four or five years just to get myself where I wanted to be with my health and I still have some kinks to work out. During the time I started on this journey, my family moved again in 2018, my daughter got married, and my son was in a serious car accident, which meant a year of my life was spent taking him to physical therapy, emotional therapy, and many other types of doctor's appointments. Life happens, but we don't have to throw in the towel! Throughout this guide I will talk about my experiences to help you see that you are not alone. Sometimes we hear stories of big successes and think "that could never be me" or "they are just naturally superhuman" or "they have extraordinary strength or will-power." The truth is that we are all unique and not one of us has the same life circumstances. But every one of us can find ways to improve and make changes. It just takes practice and perseverance to get back up and try again. I'm confident that this approach can benefit you. You can do it!

WHY THIS WORKBOOK AND BOOK?

This book and the downloadable workbook on my website are about the basics of functional medicine. The functional medicine approach is empowering because it emphasizes lifestyle, movement, and diet, all of which things we have control over. The beauty of the workbook is that, if your own detective work isn't getting you to where you want to be, you will have records that can be an extremely useful tool to help your functional health coach or doctor get you on the right track.

Using this book and workbook together can be a wonderful complement to any health plan your doctor has for you. Use the book to educate yourself and to help prepare you for answering the questions in the workbook. Use the workbook to keep track of your visits, plan of care from your doctor, as well as your own healthy lifestyle goals. Sometimes we can get caught up in a particular treatment plan and forget the basics. For instance, let's say you are working on hormone balance or treatment for Lyme disease and are focused on supplements and other treatment but are gradually forgetting stress management skills or to have some fun. That was me! This workbook can help you stay on track with those basics or help you identify some of the basics you may have been missing from the beginning.

HOW TO USE THE WORKBOOK

The workbook can be found on my website, www.function-alhealthbasics.com. You can use it in digital format or print out the pages you want when you want them. You can staple them together or add them to a binder. There are doctor's pages you can print out to take to your doctor with questions for him or her; a list of medications, supplements, and herbs you're taking; current symptoms; and other items.

What works for me is to find a good quality binder with an opening on the front and back as well as sleeves on the inside of the front and back cover. That way I can slip my current plan of care right into the front for quick access. For my binder, I have my doctor's plan of care on the front and current labs on the back. Within the inside sleeves I have informational pamphlets and papers. You can also insert plastic sleeves into the binder itself for recipes, ideas, and helpful articles you may take out of a magazine or from the Web. It's something that can be tailored to your unique circumstances.

The beauty of the workbook is that when life is topsy turvy you can put it down and pick it up again when you are ready. The benefit is that you are going to have a record of what works for you and what doesn't.

I truly hope this guide is informative and helpful on your wellness journey.

CHAPTER 1
THE FUNCTIONAL MEDICINE APPROACH

———————— ❧ ————————

WHAT IS FUNCTIONAL MEDICINE?

To get a clearer picture of what functional medicine is, let's compare it with conventional and holistic medicine, taking the treatment of fibromyalgia as an example. Conventional medicine will look at fibromyalgia as having an unknown origin and prescribe medicine and physical therapy to control the pain. Holistic practitioners may focus on specific treatments such as massage therapy, chiropractic adjustments, or homeopathic remedies, which are wonderful tools that complement functional medicine very nicely. However, functional medicine will look for the *root cause* of chronic health conditions. I like to think of it this way: a plant, tree, or shrub takes in nutrients through its roots. If the soil is depleted of its nutrients or if its root is damaged, the plant suffers. That's the way it is with the human body; if the foundation of our health, the way we were designed to thrive, is not functioning, our health and vitality suffer. One of the fundamental ways functional medicine gets at the root of a problem is through the 3 Rs:

- **Remove**: Remove what is causing the problem. For instance, nightshades like tomatoes, peppers, and potatoes can cause inflammation in some people, leading to arthritic conditions. Dairy causes inflammation leading to brain fog, chronic diarrhea, or abdominal pain.

- **Replace**: Replace what is missing or too low. The body could be lacking vitamin D and zinc, leading to low immune function. Or it could be a lack of thyroid hormone, leading to weight gain and fatigue. Vegans might be missing vitamin B12 in their diet.

- **Repair**: Repair any damage to the body. For instance, celiac disease will cause intestinal damage until the gluten is removed from the diet. Repairing the damage helps with proper nutritional absorption in the intestines and prevents leaky gut issues. The body is designed to repair itself if we give it the proper support through nutrition, stress management, and other aspects of a healthy lifestyle.

Finding the root of the problem and applying the 3 Rs can bring a person much relief. Undiagnosed nutritional deficiencies (vitamin D, magnesium, etc.) or food intolerances or sensitivities such as to nightshades or gluten are often the culprit. Perhaps stress management or past trauma are at the root of the problem. Sometimes there is an even deeper issue such as undiagnosed Lyme disease or mold exposure. Doctors of functional medicine may use medicine if needed but not before doing their due diligence as a detective. After discovering the problem, the culprit is removed, what is low or missing is replaced, and any damage is repaired.

Why did I use fibromyalgia at the beginning of the section as an example? Because that, along with hypothyroidism, were my first diagnoses in my late twenties. It wasn't until I was almost forty that I started to get accurate diagnoses, which began my search for the how and why. And here I am, healthier and functioning better than I was in my twenties, thirties, and forties.

I'm not talking about perfect health. What I am talking about is chronic health issues we have control over. Things like type-2 diabetes, heart disease, high blood pressure, chronic gut ailments, and chronic fatigue or pain. Yes, you read that right! Even though we may be genetically set up for these illnesses, science is proving that it takes triggers to set these genes into action. The CDC defines epigenetics as "the study of how our environment and behaviors can cause changes that affect how our genes work. Unlike genetic changes, epigenetic changes are reversible and do not change our DNA sequence, but they can change how our body reads a DNA sequence." When we make positive changes in our diet, environment, and stress management, we can avoid, manage, or even reverse many chronic illnesses.

7 PILLARS FOR OBTAINING OPTIMAL HEALTH

There are basically seven pillars of wellness, and we have a measure of control over each one: food, environment, stress, sleep, safe movement, fun, and awareness and appreciation of life (some call this spirituality). Each one of us has a unique approach to life based on our experiences and how we were raised. And our body type is different for each one of us. Some of these sections may be more difficult for you than your neighbor, or you may have a head start on certain area your neighbor lacks greatly in. Let's take diet, for instance. This has been my number-one biggest challenge because I came from a family that consumed a lot of boxed processed meals. Rice with seasoning came in a little carton, so there was a time I had no idea how to make rice from scratch. Candy, cake (Hostess, anyone?), cookies, and, not to forget the best of all, grandma's peanut butter fudge, were all staples when I was growing up. Uh, no wonder I come from a family of overweight diabetics with heart disease.

It did not come easy for me to learn how to cook healthily, eat vegetables, and make wise food decisions. Although I'm really not a fan of cooking, I love to bake! (And eat it all—ha-ha!) Added to that has been the challenge of having a variety of diets in my home. Some of it was because of my gluten-free diet or the twenty-plus food sensitivities my son had at one time. I could work around that, but the biggest challenge has been my husband and kids being picky and preferring familiar meals or processed and fast foods. The challenges remain, but by persevering and being creative at seeking out solutions, I have found success. Maybe you have similar challenges with your diet. Or maybe food is not a challenge for you. Perhaps you have a type-A personality and struggle with perfectionism.

Then you might find that stress management and having fun will be a challenge for you. Or maybe like me, you have a combo of challenges as you start this journey.

So as you begin this journey, step back and really think about what it is you want to accomplish. What can you manage in your life right now? Start there and perhaps dabble a little in some of the other areas. For instance, does tackling food seem a bit overwhelming? Then start where you feel more comfortable and less stressed out, maybe just adding one salad or vegetable soup a day to your menu while working on safe movement or having fun. Use the workbook to help you work through what it is you want to accomplish. With the help of this book and workbook, I know you can succeed!

CHAPTER 2

FOOD

———————————— 🌿 ————————————

Food: what does it have to do with health and wellness? Everything! Have you heard the saying, "Food can make you sick or it can make you well"? Making changes through just this one pillar of health can drastically improve your level of wellness. Let me tell you, I fought this one tooth and nail for years and eventually had to admit my diet was the biggest obstacle to my health.

Here is just a little example of my struggle with accepting this truth. Back in 2005 I visited an MD for my thyroid. I knew he tended to think outside of the box. I just wasn't feeling that great on Synthroid and I wanted something more natural. I immediately knew there was something to his way of practicing medicine when my first visit was an hour long and he considered all aspects of my health and whole-body symptoms. What I had learned in nursing school when I took anatomy and physiology was that every part of the body is connected and what affects one system can affect other systems. This is not the approach of conventional medicine. In conventional medicine there are specialists for everything and often no collaboration among them. So here I was wanting a different option for my thyroid, and after the lab results came back I ended up with two accurate diagnoses that years of going to one specialist after another didn't produce. They were Hashimoto's (an autoimmune thyroid condition) and celiac disease (an autoimmune intestinal illness). At that time my gut issues weren't even my focus. I was ignoring the constipation and abdominal pain. My lack of energy, depression, muscle pain, numbness in my legs, and overall feeling of blah were what I wanted help with.

There wasn't going to be any magic pill. The doctor told me I needed to start a gluten-free diet *and* get off sugar. Here was my mentality: I had all the laboratory proof I needed, along with the research I did on celiac disease, to come to the conclusion that yes, I needed to stop eating gluten. And I did, 100 percent. However, I was not totally convinced that abstaining from sugar was the answer for me. I didn't have diabetes or any other laboratory tests to prove to me that sugar was my nemesis. So that's how I lived my life for the next five to six years until I read *Eat to Live* by Dr. Fuhrman. It was a great eye opener about how food affects us, and I tried his diet plan for a while. It was mostly vegan—and hard. I lost a little weight, but I still didn't feel well. Then I started learning about functional medicine through Dr. Hyman and his sugar detox book. And while the sugar detox still didn't quite fit the bill for me, his book educated me on functional medicine and led me to consider an elimination diet. Gradually, I learned that certain foods were causing problems for me. These are typical, everyday foods that most people have problems with, and they just have no clue!

I finally started to eat not to lose weight but to feel better. What has been the result? I feel great and, as of this writing, I've lost almost fifty pounds! As I stated in my introduction, it still took me four to five years to implement these changes in my diet and make them a lifestyle. But now I no longer follow any particular diet plan, nor do I count calories or macronutrients. Much of my diet tends to lean towards paleo, but not 100 percent. What I have discovered along the way is how to listen to my body to know how much I can tolerate certain foods and which foods I need to still avoid like the plague.

For instance, gluten. I have to 100 percent avoid it or my body reacts violently. Grains and certain starches tend to sit in my gut. Cassava, although not a grain, is notorious for causing me to bloat. And what about my beloved cheese? On rare occasions I will have RSBT-free cheese and can tolerate it just fine. But there is a line and if I cross it, I will have gut issues and nasal congestion. But dairy in general I avoid. What about sugar, another one of my much-loved foods? On the weekends, I will have a small treat made from grains and sugar. I don't dare bake, as I will eat it all. Ha-ha! Instead of baking, I will buy something small or something that my family likes so they can help me eat it. It keeps life simple and food enjoyable.

I approach food as a lifestyle so I eat to nourish my body and to feel well. But I still set up a time to look forward to a moment of tasty gratification. Why? Because life is meant to be enjoyed. I know, I know, you will hear experts on sugar

I JUST WANT TO FUNCTION!

detox tell you it's just like an alcoholic: the addiction is so bad that just one time will cause you to fall off the ladder. True enough . . . especially at first. But, what happens when you go to that party after you have been off sugar for so long and have a piece of cake? You lose control! I found out that if I set a time to have a sweet treat, then I don't feel deprived and it's easier to stick with eating healthily. The key, however, is to do a sugar detox to reset your system. Once you do that, you will see how much better you feel off of sugar and then you might decide that a little here or there won't be a problem for you. Listen to your body and make the best decision for you and reevaluate as time goes by.

Fortunately, there are easy-to-follow elimination diets out there to help you to come to the answers pretty quickly. Elimination diets eliminate foods known to cause a variety of health reactions, whether outright or subtle. Often, people will be having a reaction to a food without being aware of it. After eliminating the food for a time and then adding it back, a reaction will occur if that person has a sensitivity. The Whole 30 Diet and The AIP (Autoimmune Protocol) are just two examples. What do these approaches have in common and why do so many people find relief when they do an elimination diet? It's because the top inflammatory foods are eliminated: gluten (grains in general), dairy, soy, processed foods, and sugar. These diets also add in plenty of healing foods that nourish our bodies in harmony with the way we are designed.

Use this chapter as a tool to listen to what your body is trying to tell you. Doing a full elimination diet may be too overwhelming for you. If so, then just pick one thing at a time to eliminate, or you could set a goal to replace one meal a day with a salad, vegetable soup, or smoothie that includes protein and a healthy fat. You may be so sick of feeling sick that you want to do a deep dive right into doing a full elimination diet. That's great! In fact, I recommend it, because then you can feel crummy for about a week with the withdrawals and detoxifying effects, but after that you will see how great you feel in just a short period of time. When you start to add food back in, you will be clearer on how each food will make you feel. It's a much faster process than one food at a time, and it's very possible that it's more than one food that is causing you troubles. On my website, I have links to resources that will take you to a variety of options that can guide you on your journey.

(Note: before you begin any dietary change, talk with your doctor first.)

INFLAMMATORY FOODS

Let's talk a little bit about the top foods (grains, gluten, dairy, soy, sugar, and ultra-processed) that cause inflammation and why. Inflammation is an immune response to something the body views as harmful. This response can be localized in the case of an injury or infection, or it can be body wide in the case of a variety of factors such as food sensitivities or stress. Learning about inflammatory foods can help you to make a more informed choice of where to start if you choose not to do a full-fledged elimination diet. (To learn more about inflammation, including what it is and why it's important to reduce or eliminate, see chapter 12).

GRAINS

Back in 2005, I totally removed wheat, rye, and barley (gluten-containing grains) from my diet because I had been diagnosed with celiac disease. It wasn't until 2016 that I removed all grains from my diet, which proved to be the most helpful in my health. That was when my gut started to fully feel normal and I really started to steadily drop the weight. Most people tolerate gluten-free whole grains just fine. However, some of the same problems exist with most grains as they do with gluten-containing grains. The way grains are processed is very different in today's world compared to the past. Grains used to be soaked, sprouted, and fermented so that they could be easily digested. This also preserved the germ, fiber, and vital nutrients. Our bodies were designed to assimilate foods as close to nature as possible, so our modern way of processing causes trouble for many people. Dr. Hyman says in his book *Food*,

> *New hybrids have been developed, most notably dwarf wheat, which is heartier than its predecessors but contains a "superstarch" called amylopectin A that has a greater impact on our blood sugar than the traditional kinds of starch—it actually promotes insulin resistance. The new varieties also have more gluten, which is not doing us any favors. And while most wheat isn't genetically modified, it is dosed with*

a chemical herbicide called glyphosate just before harvest,
which increases its yield . . . The EPA says it's safe for us,
but there's evidence suggesting it may have something to do
with the rise in celiac disease and other gluten sensitivities.
(See his book under Grains for scientific references.)

This isn't the only problem with grains. Have you seen the commercials about the lawsuits regarding Roundup containing glyphosate? As of this writing, although litigation is ongoing, Bayer has agreed to pay a settlement of 10.9 billion dollars to thousands of plaintiffs and 2 billion to future plaintiffs. But has this chemical been banned like it has been in Europe? No! It's out there in abundance. Glyphosate leads to inflammation. It's something to consider, especially if you have celiac or other autoimmune conditions.

WHAT ARE GRAINS AND HOW ARE THEY BEST EATEN?

The usual grains in our society are wheat, corn, rice, rye, oats, and barley as well as unusual grains that haven't been altered much by man such as quinoa, amaranth, buckwheat (this is not a wheat product and thus does not contain gluten), teff, and millet. We've already discussed the gluten-containing grains wheat, rye, and barley and why you need to avoid them. The rest of the grains are best eaten soaked, sprouted, and in whole organic form to preserve the nutrients and natural qualities that allow for easy digestion. Grains in such forms are not easy to find in our society and eliminating grains that are not in these forms is why many people start to feel great when starting on a paleo or keto diet!

Beware of breads that say whole grain or ancient grains as these breads are still mostly flour and act as sugar, quickly spiking blood sugar. Most often they contain very little whole grain.

GLUTEN

Gluten is a protein derived from grains like wheat, rye, and barley. Gluten is also known as the "glue" that makes baked goods hold together. As you read in the portion of this book about grains, there is evidence suggesting that the genetic modification of grains is linked to the rise in celiac disease and gluten sensitivity. Gluten sensitivities are linked to other autoimmune conditions like Hashimoto's thyroiditis. (To learn more about thyroid conditions and gluten, read chapter 16.) Because of that, it's very important to consider whether gluten is a problem for you if you have Hashimoto's or another autoimmune condition.

Many think that symptoms of gluten sensitivities or celiac are just gut related, but they are not. Here is just a short list of symptoms to look out for:

- Depression
- Headaches
- Skin eruptions
- Stomach pain
- Joint and muscle pain
- Sleep disturbance

- Inability to ward off colds or flu
- Autoimmune diseases —thyroid, lupus, rheumatoid arthritis, etc.
- Bipolar disorder
- Gluten ataxia, which is a loss of cognitive function similar to Alzheimer's or dementia.

What to look for when avoiding gluten: First and foremost, choose whole foods that are not grains, like vegetables, fruits, meats, and nuts, and that are in their natural form or close to it. Shopping the perimeter of the grocery store is where you will find these foods. When it comes to boxed, processed foods, the ultimate option is for the product to be certified gluten free. If it's not, look for these ingredients to avoid:

- Wheat
- Wheat berries
- Durum
- Emmer
- Semolina
- Spelt
- Farina
- Farro
- Graham
- Kamut wheat
- Einhorn wheat
- Bulgur
- Rye
- Barley
- Triticale
- Malt
- Brewer's yeast
- Triticum vulgare
- Hordeum vulgare
- Secale cereale
- Triticum spelt
- Couscous
- Seitan

These ingredients may contain gluten (check with the manufacturer):

- Vegetable protein/hydrolyzed vegetable protein
- Modified starch/modified food starch
- Natural flavoring
- Artificial flavor
- Hydrolyzed plant protein
- "Seasonings" containing wheat filler
- Vegetable starch
- Dextrin and maltodextrin
- Oats (Look for certified gluten free. Bob's Red Mill has a certified gluten free option)

DAIRY

Dairy is one of the top-eight allergens that are required to be listed on food labels by the FDA for obvious allergic reactions. However, did you know that dairy can cause many other reactions or illnesses that are not obvious?

THE PROBLEMS WITH DAIRY:

- Just like many grains, dairy is not what it used to be. Cows are bred and raised to mass produce milk, causing it to be much different than true quality milk.

- Milk is full of hormones that promote the growth of the baby. No matter the species, the milk was designed for the growth of *that* species. Humans are the only species that choose to drink milk past infancy and not human milk! While eaten in moderation, cheese and other dairy products can be a wonderful treat, but consider whether dairy should be a regular, daily part of your diet.

- Some of the hormones in dairy have been found to be linked to cancer. Take IGF-1 (insulin growth factor), for instance, which is known to cause cancer and has been linked to heart disease and type-2 diabetes.

- Milk from cows contains several different allergens; one in particular is casein. Casein has been linked to eczema, ear infections, congestion, and sinus problems.

- Most adults no longer have the enzyme lactase to break down the milk protein lactose, which leads to stomach upset, bloating, and gas, which are indications of whole-body inflammation.

If you choose to avoid dairy, where can you start? Because dairy is one of the top-eight allergens that must be listed on food packaging as an ingredient in the US, reading labels will be very useful in knowing if the product contains dairy. Finding dairy-free options for milk products is easier than ever in today's market. There are a variety of nuts, rice, coconut, oat milk, and other dairy-free milks to choose from. Yogurts have dairy-free versions as well. With all these options you should have no problem finding a replacement you aren't sensitive to.

SOY

Soy, like dairy, is also listed as one of the top allergens that has to be listed on labels as such. That means the US government has determined that it is one of the top-eight foods individuals are allergic to. Allergy and sensitivity are two different things, and many proponents of a healthy diet will list soy as a health food. Unfortunately, our modern soy leaves much to be desired when it comes to health. Apart from soy being among the top-eight allergens, here are some more valid reasons for avoiding soy if you find you are dealing with chronic health concerns:

- Much of the soy grown today has been genetically modified. As we learned earlier, GMOs can be unrecognizable by the body as a fully usable food source.

- Soy is phytoestrogenic. The plants naturally produce a pesticide called isoflavone to protect it from insects. Many proponents of soy's place in a healthy diet will say that isoflavones are good for you. However, isoflavones are estrogen-like compounds linked to a variety of disease processes. This phytoestrogenic property is seen by the body as an estrogen. Why is this a problem? Because many people deal with estrogen dominance, which in turn causes the liver to produce excessive thyroid-binding globulin, leading to low thyroid activity. This is especially important to consider for those who have thyroid problems.

- There are hundreds of studies linking soy to a variety of other disease processes, including heart disease and cancer.

What ingredients do you need to avoid if you are going to give soy elimination a try?

- Many processed foods. If you are buying processed boxed or canned foods, the label will state that it contains soy. So look for that statement within or under the ingredients list.

- Soy or teriyaki sauce is an obvious place where you will find soy. A good replacement for soy sauce is coconut aminos, which is just as delicious.

- Tofu, miso, natto, and tempeh.

- High-protein energy bars or powders. Again, check the labels.

- Meat substitutes (often reads as textured vegetable protein TVP).

- Products that list glycine max, hydrolyzed protein (HVP), mono-diglyceride, or monosodium glutamate.

- Edamame.

SUGAR

Who doesn't love a nice sweet treat? Remember in the beginning of this book I mentioned my grandmother's homemade peanut butter fudge? I remember my mom making it when I was young, and in the middle of the night I would go into the cupboard while everyone was asleep and sneak off with some. That's how much I loved it! Did my parents ever wonder where all that fudge went? Hee-hee!

In 2015, when we were on the go all the time because of moving, I fell into the trap of grabbing a sixteen-ounce Pepsi every day just to get that little boost of energy. That led me to going down to the gas station daily because I refused to buy it with groceries and have it in the house. I knew it was a bad dietary choice, so I purposely made it harder for myself. But when I went to the gas station, usually in the morning, for that Pepsi, sugar, and caffeine fix, I didn't stop with just a Pepsi; I would also buy a Snickers or other candy I was craving. I knew I was acting like an addict. And I was acting like an addict because I *was* an addict! One of the biggest problems with refined, processed, sugary snacks is their addictiveness. Some experts believe it is worse than cocaine in the way that it acts on the brain. So why be concerned with wanting to eat excess sugary foods? There are several reasons, and I'll go through them one at a time.

- **Inflammation**. Too much sugar is inflammatory. One way sugar causes inflammation is by disrupting the microbial balance in the gut, leading to a leaky gut or SIBO (Small Intestinal Bacterial Overgrowth). When the gut is out of balance (also called dysbiosis) it can become inflamed, leading to cramping, diarrhea, or constipation. This dysbiosis in the gut can also cause nutritional deficiencies that affect the ability of the immune system to function properly, which can trigger body-wide inflammation. Some autoimmune responses and fibromyalgia are linked to a diet high in sugar.

- **Obesity and type-2 diabetes**. You may have heard that eating too much fat can make you fat, but the truth is that sugar is far more likely to play a role in the body's desire to store fat. The higher our diet is in sugar, the more impact the pancreas is disrupted in its ability to produce insulin. Insulin takes the blood sugar and stores it for energy to use later on. This is the natural process our bodies use to turn glucose into energy so we can thrive. Unfortunately, when we consume way more sugar than the body was designed to need, the various cells that store sugar for energy to use later on are desensitized and stop responding to the insulin cues. This leads to the glucose being stored as fat and we gain weight. Eventually, for many this will lead to type-2 diabetes.

- **Other impacts of a high-sugar diet**. A diet high in sugar has been linked to thyroid problems and nervous system disorders such as anxiety, depression, brain fog, and inability to manage stress. It has also been linked to hormone imbalances, lower immunity, disrupted sleep and menstrual cycles, as well as cancer.

WHAT CAN YOU DO TO LOWER YOUR REFINED SUGAR INTAKE?

- Swap high-sugar treats for fruit, which is full of blood-sugar regulating fiber and better processed by the body. (If you are diabetic, please talk with your healthcare provider about any changes you make with your diet.)

- Since our bodies need sugar to function properly, look for healthier, natural varieties of sugar like fruits, honey, or maple syrup to use in moderation. Stevia is a good sugar substitute as well.

- Look for a good anti-inflammatory diet that will help your whole body heal from the chronic inflammation that it may be dealing with. A few that I recommend are the one detailed in Dr. Hyman's book *The Blood Sugar Solution 10-Day Detox Diet Cookbook*, The Autoimmune Protocol (AIP Diet), or any anti-inflammatory diet that seems good for you.

RESOURCES:

- Michael Moss (*New York Times* reporter), *Salt Sugar Fat: How the Food Giants Hooked Us*

- Dr. Hyman, *The Blood Sugar Solution 10-Day Detox Diet*

PROCESSED FOODS

Most foods in our society are processed to one degree or another. Processing is when a food product is altered from its natural state and can range from minimally processed to ultra-processed. You may be interested to know that there are over 15,000 chemicals in our food supply. Most of these chemicals have never been tested for safety in the Unites States and some are banned in other countries because of the known harm they cause. We live in a fast-paced society and for most it's not practical or even possible to totally avoid processed foods entirely. So let's discuss what processed foods even are and what it is we want to totally avoid or, at best, decrease in our diet.

Minimally processed foods are foods that are processed for the purpose of preservation and shipment. These are foods that are cleaned up, ground up, fermented, refrigerated, frozen, bagged up, or pasteurized. In general, this category still mostly contains whole foods you buy at the store. For example, fresh kale tied up in a bunch or bagged and frozen green beans would fall into this category. Then there are whole foods that are processed a bit further by adding other ingredients like salt, sugar, and fats. Example of this would be a bag of frozen, microwave-ready green beans with added salt and butter. Foods in this category are easily identified by their ingredients. The biggest concern with these products is the amount of salt and the addition of unhealthy fats or refined sugar. Ultra-processed foods are loaded with all kinds of additives with unpronounceable words on the labels, which we will get into further in the chapter.

I've already talked about sugar at length and why you want to lower your intake of it. Now we are going to dive into salt and fats that may be processed themselves and are found in processed foods. You may be surprised that I will tell you to eat salt and fat because they are important for the body. However, there are some cautions you need to be aware of.

- Salt is necessary for survival and good health. We need it for proper electrolyte balance in our bodies and electrolyte replacement for those who sweat a lot. In general, though, it is a good idea to eat salt in moderation and just be aware of excess intake as that can be inflammatory. The biggest concern with salt intake would be for those who have a health condition where a doctor has prescribed a low-salt diet. Here is a very informative article on salt that really dives into the origin of salt, consumption differences in other cultures, as well as types of salt: *https://chriskresser.com/specialreports/salt/*

- Fat is also necessary for our survival and good health because we need it for proper cellular, mental, and hormonal function in the body. The low-fat trends of the past years have only contributed to disease and weight gain because when the food producers removed the fats from foods, they increased the salt, sugar, and other food additives to maintain the flavor of their food. When I started including fat in my diet, I not only started to feel better, I also was able to finally start losing weight. Granted, adding fat in my diet wasn't the sole magic bullet that benefited me, but my body was getting the fats it needed to work properly. Fat in general is not the enemy. Bad fats are. These fats contain omega-6 fats that can be very inflammatory whereas, omega-3 fats are the opposite: they are anti-inflammatory. There is a lot to be said about fat, but to make it simple I'll list the types of fats to avoid and the types of fat to consume. If you want to know more, these great articles go into depth about fats.

https://chriskresser.com/healthy-fats-what-you-need-to-know/
https://experiencelife.lifetime.life/video/a-conversation-with
 -dr-mark-hyman-video/

- Get healthy fats from coconut oil, organic cold-pressed olive oil, avocado oil, grass-fed butter and ghee (if you tolerate dairy), walnut oil, pecan oil, and flaxseed.

- Eat whole foods that are full of healthy fats such as nuts, seeds, nut and seed butters, avocados, olives, wild fatty fish, and eggs. (If you have no known allergy or sensitivity any of these foods.)

- Avoid or restrict refined oils like vegetable, corn, soybean, sunflower, canola, peanut, grapeseed, and safflower oil.

The types of processed foods we should really be concerned with, especially if you are struggling with chronic health concerns, is ultra-processed foods. Ultra-processed foods contain artificial food colorings and flavorings, pre-servatives, and ingredients to preserve texture and flavor. Many of these foods are low in nutrients and fiber but full of calories, sugar, salt, unhealthy fats, and chemicals, thus leading to many chronic health problems, obesity, and inflammation. We've already talked about sugar, salt, and unhealthy fats so now we will talk about all the other additives that may be concerning to you.

One rule of thumb with processed foods is that if you must eat processed foods (and, as I noted above, they're hard to avoid completely) try to choose ones that are as minimally processed as possible. The smaller the ingredient list, the better the food may be. A good source of information is Environmental Working Group's (EWG's) list of dirty dozen food additives to avoid.

https://www.ewg.org/consumer-guides/ewgs-dirty-dozen-guide-food-additives

Here are some additives you would really want to consider avoiding and why:

- **Artificial sweeteners**: This type of additive includes sucralose, aspartame, and sugar alcohols such as maltitol, sorbitol, isomalt, and erythritol. These artificial sweeteners have been shown to contribute to impaired glucose tolerance and affect the balance of the gut, leading to weight gain and a lower metabolism. If you need to use a sugar substitute try the more natural alternatives like stevia and monk fruit.

- **Monosodium glutamate (MSG)**: This can be hidden on the labels as "vegetable protein," "hydrolyzed vegetable protein (HVP)," "natural flavorings," and "spices." Making the name sound harmless is how the food companies hide it from consumers. But what is wrong with MSG in the first place? It's an excitotoxin that negatively affects brain cells and increases hunger and carb cravings.

- **High fructose corn syrup (HFCS)**: It is well known that HFCS is inflammatory and has been linked to obesity, weight gain, diabetes, heart disease, fatty liver disease, cancer, and dementia. HFCS has absolutely no nutritional benefit and is empty calories. Is your health worth risking just for the tasty benefits of daily consumption?

- **Nitrates or nitrites**: Nitrates and nitrites occur naturally in our environment and in many foods yet by adding them to processed meats and other foods can have negative effects on our bodies, including cancer.
  https://www.ncbi.nlm.nih.gov/pmc/articles/PMC7139399/

- **Other additives that may be linked to cancer, endocrine disruptions, or other health concerns:** Many of these are banned in Canada, the United Kingdom, and the European Union; they include propyl gallate, butylated hydoxytoluene (BHT), butylated hydroxyanisole (BHA), propylparaben, and potassium bromate.

- **Artificial colorings**: They have been linked to many negative health consequences like hypersensitivity and cancer.

- **Artificial flavorings**: They may even say "natural flavorings," which can contain undisclosed BHT or propylene glycol.

SUMMARY: THE BEST DIETARY CHOICES

Whether you choose to eliminate certain foods to see if they are affecting your health or not, an optimal diet will be balanced and full of natural whole foods. On a daily basis, eat as many colorful non-starchy vegetables as you want, a good portion of healthy proteins, and a moderate amount of whole grains, fruits, and healthy fats such as nuts, nut butters, olive oil, and coconut oil. This way you will get plenty of nutrients and fiber to promote an overall healthy body. Eat sweets and drink alcohol sparingly. Consider setting aside just one day each week to have that cookie, candy, or cake. It will give you something to look forward to without feeling deprived.

If you've decided that an elimination diet is a route you would like to take, here are some good quality plans that you might consider:

- The Whole 30

- The AIP (Autoimmune Protocol)

- The Elimination Diet (by Alissa Segersten and Tom Malterre, MS, CN)

- Another diet your functional medicine practitioner recommends

CHAPTER 3

ENVIRONMENTAL TOXINS

———————— ༒ ————————

Let's face it, we live in a very toxic world. From air pollution to pesticides in our food, we can't escape. Some of us are like the canaries in coal mines that warned the workers of toxic gases. If the canaries started dying, the miners knew to get out. Most of us aren't dying of toxic exposure but some of us are very sensitive and are sick because our detox pathways aren't as efficient as others. Some have chronic health problems and don't even realize their environment is the source. Thankfully, there is much we can do to lower our toxic exposure. In this section, I'm going to discuss the ways we are exposed to toxins, why it matters to our health and well-being, and what we can do about lowering our exposure. Pick just one thing to work on and add more as you can. Feeling stressed can be a big factor in our well-being as you will see in the next chapter. So do what you can one step at a time. Little changes can bring benefits.

FOOD

In previous chapters I've talked about food in depth. Outside of breathing, food is one of the easiest ways to increase our toxic exposure. So you may be thinking, "More food restrictions?" or "Won't this be expensive?" Now, hear me out: if you are already making changes with your food choices based on my chapter on foods, this should be a piece of cake. (Never mind the pun, ha-ha!) The most important thing is to be aware and find ways to lower your exposure. Even if it's just a little at a time, you can still feel good about it.

PESTICIDES AND PRODUCE

Have you seen the commercials about glyphosate (Roundup)? If you want to see how prevalent this problem is, do an internet search for "glyphosate map." Some of them will show the increased use in just the past decade or two. Why should we be worried about glyphosate? It has been confirmed by many scientists, physicians around the world, as well as US and international government agencies that the potential health risks of glyphosate and other pesticides include brain and nervous system toxicity (anxiety, Parkinson's), cancer, hormone disruption (in particular, hypothyroidism), and suppressed immune system. Another herbicide of concern is 2,4-D, and these are just two of many. So what can you do to lower your exposure?

Some people may choose to go completely organic, and that's great for those who can afford it. What if going completely organic is just not doable for you? That's okay! It's better to eat produce that has some pesticides on it than to avoid it completely. That's because produce is chock full of nutrients that the body needs to thrive. To keep costs down and minimize pesticide intake, you can eat from both categories. Some fruits and vegetables are much higher in pesticides than others, so try to choose organic versions so you can lower your exposure and at the same time keep your grocery bill at a more affordable level. An example of this is strawberries and apples. Both are notorious for having a high level of pesticides. You can choose to eat those organic while eating pineapple and cantaloupe conventionally grown. The Environmental Working Group has a list of the "Dirty Dozen" that shows which produce still has the highest pesticides *after washing them* (these would be the ones to eat organically) and a list of the "Clean 15" that shows the least toxic produce. I've included these lists here, but for more information and updates go to www.EWG.org. You can feel good about eating conventionally grown produce from the Clean 15 without worries about heavy pesticides and then take extra precautions with the produce from the Dirty Dozen, eating them organic whenever possible.

DIRTY DOZEN: EAT ORGANIC IF POSSIBLE

- Strawberries
- Spinach
- Kale
- Nectarines
- Apples
- Grapes
- Peaches
- Cherries
- Pears
- Tomatoes
- Celery
- Potatoes

CLEAN 15: PRODUCE WITH THE
LEAST PESTICIDE RESIDUES

- Avocados
- Sweet corn*
- Pineapple
- Onions
- Papaya*
- Sweet peas, frozen
- Eggplant
- Asparagus
- Cauliflower
- Cantaloupe
- Broccoli
- Mushrooms
- Cabbage
- Honeydew melon
- Kiwi

*A small amount of these crops are produced from genetically modified seeds (GMOs). Buy organic varieties of these if you want to avoid GMOs.

GMOS

Beyond pesticides, many foods have been genetically modified for a variety of reasons. For instance, field corn and soy grown in the United States are genetically modified to withstand applications of Roundup and sometimes 2,4-D (as mentioned, another herbicide with known health risks). Some may be concerned about man redesigning what was originally found in nature. Is this what our bodies were designed to digest and assimilate? What are the long-term repercussions? For these reasons, a person may want to avoid GMOs. The easiest way to do this is to buy organic. Organic foods are non-GMO. Look for the green USDA Organic label or the "Non-GMO Project Verified" label.

MERCURY AND FISH

By now the whole scientific community is on board with how dangerous mercury is to the body, at least to some degree. According to the WHO (World Health Organization), "mercury—even in small amounts—may cause serious health problems and is a threat to the development of the unborn child and in early life. Mercury may have toxic effects on the nervous, digestive, and immune systems, and on the lungs, kidneys, skin, and eyes." The WHO also considers mercury to be one of the top-ten chemicals of public concern.

High levels of mercury can be found in fish. The bigger the fish, the larger the levels of mercury. Fish is a good source of healthy omega-3 fatty acids that reduce inflammation, support a healthy cardiovascular system, and help with anxiety and depression. Because fish in general is good for us, the safest fish to eat are smaller, wild-caught fish like salmon and sardines. There are some brands of canned tuna that are labeled as safe. If you like some of the bigger fish, consider eating them only on occasion and try increasing the amounts of safer fish in your diet. Here is a good resource for choosing which fish to eat: *https://www.epa.gov/fish-tech/ epa-fda-advice-about-eating-fish-and-shellfish*

AIR QUALITY

Outside: The type of toxins in the outdoor air depends on where you live. In cities or communities where there are industrial businesses, you may be exposed to different toxins than if you were living around farmland. Even suburban neighborhoods have their own toxins. I just happen to live in a townhome community and they spray the lawn frequently, which not only affects us but also my neighbors who live nearby because it just drifts over to their property. There are a very few places left where exposure to toxins is low.

TIPS FOR KEEPING THESE OUTDOOR TOXINS FROM GETTING INSIDE YOUR HOME

- Close windows and run the air on days when chemical spraying occurs, whether it's from farms or lawns.

- Make sure you wipe your pets off when they come indoors. We just walk our dog at the park for a few days after they spray.

- Take your shoes off at the door.

- Buy a good quality HEPA air purifier. Two brands I recommend are Austin and IQAir.

- For city and suburb dwellers, close windows on bad air quality days and run the air purifier.

Inside: The indoor pollution in the home is often worse than it is outside. It is estimated that the air inside is two to five times more polluted than the air outside. See www.EWG. org/healthyhomeguide for more in-depth information. In the meantime, here is a basic breakdown of what could be lurking in your indoor air, why it is dangerous, and some simple steps to improve air quality:

- VOCs (volatile organic compounds) are known to cause asthma attacks or irritate the nose and eyes. One VOC, formaldehyde, is known to cause cancer. Cleaning supplies, scented candles, fragrances, and scented personal care products all contain VOCs that harm our bodies.

- PVCs (polyvinyl chloride) is considered by some to be the most toxic plastic because it is made from vinyl chloride, which is a cancerous product. Some flexible PVCs have phthalates in them, which are known endocrine (hormone) disruptors.

- PFCs (perfluorinated chemicals) found in nonstick cookware, carpets, and waterproof clothing accumulate in the body and cause hormone disruption, weakened immune systems, and possibly cancer.

- Antimicrobials (antibacterial and anti-mold)—added to carpets, countertops, paints, engineered wood, and ceiling tiles—can cause harm. Triclosan, for instance, is an endocrine disruptor.

- PBDEs (flame retardants), found in fabrics, foam, and electronics, are associated with endocrine disruption, immunotoxicity, and cancer. They have also been linked to problems with the nervous system and fetal development.

- Lead and asbestos are no longer used in building materials and paints because of their known serious health risks but are still found in older homes.

- Radon is an odorless gas that can cause lung cancer. It can leak into the home from the soil.

What can you do? Maybe you just put carpeting in, not knowing what you know now. Maybe you just put in countertops that contain an antimicrobial agent. For these things, check out www. EWG.org/healthyhomeguide for tips to remain healthy now and make better choices in the future. For some of the smaller changes you can make now, here is a list of what to consider:

- Stop using air fresheners and scented candles.*

- Stop using cleaning or laundry products that list "fragrance" as an ingredient without stating what exactly that fragrance ingredient is. Many fragrances contain suspected endocrine (hormone) disruptors like phthalates and can cause breathing problems.*

- Buy an air purifier to help lower the toxic load from the off-gassing of the furnishings in your home. There are special air purifiers that will filter out VOCs. Both IQAir and Austin have such filters.

- Consider buying furniture that is used and has off-gassed much of the chemicals. You will be amazed at what you can find through various resale options. You can also feel good about being environmentally conscious.

- If you live in an older home and you plan on doing some remodeling, have it inspected by a certified professional for asbestos before demolishing.

- Always check for radon before you buy a home during your home inspection. If you haven't moved in a long time and want to check for radon in your own home, there are easy-to-use kits found in hardware stores to detect the presence.

- Wash new clothes and bedding before use.

- Consider switching from plastics to glass or ceramic containers a little at a time.

- Ditch the nonstick cookware and use cast iron, stainless steel, or ceramic. This is because many of the chemicals listed previously are in the nonstick cookware and are released into the air when the pot or pan is heated.

- Choose one room at a time to make as toxin free as possible. Start with the bedrooms because you spend a third of your life there, and while you are sleeping you are breathing deeply.

*If you really enjoy fragrances, choose essential oils that are 100-percent pure, therapeutic grade. The reason is that the essential oil industry is largely unregulated. Many cheap essential oils can be labeled 100-percent pure and only have a small percentage of that essential oil or even synthetic "essential oil" in it. What else is in that bottle of essential oil? Who knows? But they are cheap for a reason! Good quality essential oils use a lot of plant material to obtain the genuine oil and can be costly to extract, which is why they are more expensive. You know good quality when you see that the price of orange essential oil is different than that of rose essential oil, for example.

A Word of Caution: Some individuals have asthma or other respiratory concerns, so if that is you, ease into the use of essential oils. Some people even say they can breathe better because of essential oils! If you are reacting from good quality essential oils then it may be that your body is overloaded from the toxic chemicals that you've been using. It will take some time for your body to detox and adjust.

OTHER INDOOR POLLUTANTS:

Mold: Mold can range from a harmless little spot in the shower to toxic black mold. Toxic mold can be extremely harmful. If you suspect toxic mold could be lurking in your home, here are some good websites for help, or you could do an internet search for "Chris Kresser mold."

- *www.survivingmold.com*

- *https://daveasprey.com/my-flood-story-and-what-to-do-about-mold/*

- A great documentary to watch on YouTube is *Moldy*.

- *Note:* If you have Lyme disease you could be even more sensitive to mold in general. So following some of these protocols will be beneficial to you even if you aren't affected by toxic mold.

- **Dust**: Don't you feel like it never goes away? It's a good idea to dust regularly. If you have allergies like me, you might want to wear a mask while you dust and vacuum to keep the symptoms at bay. Cover your mattress and pillows in dust mite allergy covers and wash your sheets at least every other week to get a good night's sleep. Even if you don't have allergies, it would still be wise to try not to kick up too much dust when you clean. Many of the harmful chemicals I listed before can settle in with the dust.

- **Pollen**: If you have allergies, it would be wise to keep the windows closed on high-pollen days and run your air purifier. I have a pup I need to wipe down when she comes in from outside or else I'm miserable if I want to cuddle with her. Wash your hair before you go to bed as well, otherwise you will be sleeping in pollen.

PERSONAL CARE PRODUCTS

Most people go about their day without realizing that everything they put onto their skin is absorbed into the body. Have you noticed labels that say phthalate free or paraben free? That's because many of these ingredients are harmful to the body. Some bioaccumulate over time, building up the toxic load of the body. Maybe not at first, but gradually they build up and then they cause illness that you would never suspect came from your lotion or cologne. Phthalates, for instance, as we've already discussed, are linked to endocrine disruption. So what exactly is an endocrine disruptor? The endocrine system in the body regulates hormones. So phthalates could be a contributing factor to diabetes, thyroid dysfunction, sexual dysfunction, and adrenal issues that potentially contribute to anxiety, chronic fatigue, and other conditions.

Here is a list of common, potentially toxic, ingredients found in personal care products:

- Triclocarban: potential endocrine disruptor

- Triclosan: endocrine disruption, organ system toxicity, immune toxicity

- Formaldehyde (known under other names as well): known human carcinogen (cancer causing), immune toxic

- Toluene: human developmental toxicant

- Dibutyl phthalate (DBP): endocrine disruptor, potential respiratory toxicant

- PEG: Often combined with undisclosed chemicals such as ethylene oxide and 1,4 dioxane which have been linked to cancer. PEG also enhances absorption of other compounds that may or may not be toxic.

- Parabens: propyl, isopropyl, butyl, isobutyl: endocrine disruptors, causes of potential cellular level changes, skin toxicant

- Oxybenzone: potential endocrine disruptor, photoallergen (increased reaction when exposed to the sun)

- Diazolidinyl urea and imidazolidinyl urea: known toxicant or allergen

- "Fragrance" (actual ingredients not disclosed): potential endocrine disruptor, potential respiratory toxicant and allergen, skin toxicant, and allergen

Tip: Take it one step at a time, one product at a time because switching all of your products all at once can get pricey and stressful. Don't stress yourself out over it because stress can be just as damaging to the body. When you run out of a product, do a little investigating and choose another. First check your products out on EWG.org/skindeep* to see where they fall in the range of toxicity. If it's high on the list, switch it out for something less toxic.

*Just a heads up: as of this writing, the EWG app was not nearly as user friendly as the website. So I suggest sticking with the website.

DRINKING WATER

Did you know you can live weeks without food but only a few days without water? Water is essential for living and can be beneficial for helping the kidneys expel toxins from our bodies. Depending on how much you weigh and how much you exercise, an adult should drink between 70 to 170 ounces a day. Add twelves ounces to your daily total if you exercise thirty minutes a day. Do an internet search for a water intake calculator to see how much you need. Likely more than you anticipated. That said, consider the importance of how clean and safe your water is.

TAP WATER

If you have tap water from a city or county source it's regulated by the EPA in the United States and other governmental regulators in other countries. Referring to the United States, EWG states (based on their Tap Water Database—2019 Update) that "in almost twenty years, the EPA has not added any new contaminants to the toxic chemicals covered by the Safe Drinking Water Act." "The inexcusable failure of the federal government's responsibility to protect public health means there are no legal limits for more than 160 unregulated contaminants in U.S. tap water. For some other chemicals, the EPA's Maximum Contaminant Levels, or MCLs, haven't been updated in almost fifteen years." The article goes on to state that many of these unregulated agricultural and industrial chemicals are linked to cancer, neurological damage, developmental and fertility problems, as well as hormone disruption. And this is the water that you thought was safe!

WELL WATER

If you have well water, consider the surrounding farmlands or, in some towns, industrial plants. Many potential chemicals may be leaching into your water from those sources, not to mention other contaminants from lawn care or buried/spilled chemicals from years past.

WHAT CAN YOU DO?

First look up www.EWG.org/tapwater and learn more. On their menu you will see a "Water Filter Guide" option. The best filtering option is a reverse osmosis system. However, be aware that it will also filter out important nutrients like calcium and magnesium. These nutrients are essential, and with an added filter or water drops those minerals can be added back in.

SUMMARY

We live in a very toxic world. Whether it's from the food we eat, the air we breathe, or the water we drink, toxins are everywhere. The good news is that our bodies were designed to detoxify. The bad news is that there's a limit to the amount and type of toxins our bodies can detoxify. By lowering our exposure in the areas we have control over, we increase our ability to be healthy and feel vibrant.

CHAPTER 4

STRESS

———————— ❧ ————————

What is life without stress? In fact, to a degree our bodies are designed to effectively manage short-term stress. However, with modern-day life it seems like there's never an end to stress. This isn't good for our bodies and it could be the root cause of many chronic health problems. Why? If the body is in a constant stressed-out state, our adrenals are working overtime. The adrenals are hormone-producing glands on top of our kidneys that regulate metabolism, the immune system, blood pressure, and our response to stress. When your body is always reacting to stressors, you constantly feel like you are under attack; this is the fight-or-flight reaction. Long-term, over-exposure to cortisol and other stress hormones disrupts how your body works and leads to chronic health problems like anxiety, depression, digestive problems, headaches, heart disease, sleep issues, weight gain, memory problems, and difficulty concentrating. Having said that, life is just stressful! So how can we manage? This chapter is about learning to manage how we perceive stress and healthy ways to deal with it.

I didn't even know what stress management was until my son was in a DBT (Dialectical Behavior Therapy) program. I just thought meditation in the stress-release sense was emptying your mind. Little did I know that there are many tools one can use to help reduce and manage stress.

First, we need to look at ourselves.

- Are you asking too much of yourself? Do you tend to want everything done perfectly? Do you tend to take on too much that you have a hard time managing life? Do you have a hard time saying no to others?

- Are you living today's life or are you looking back, not being able to let go of past mistakes or problems with others? Are you looking forward with dread, worried about the future, and thinking of the worst-case scenarios?

- Are you easily distracted? I recently read an article in *Experience Magazine* where the author calls the easily distracted mind the "monkey brain." Watch monkeys and you will get it, especially if, like me, you have this problem.

- Do you spend a lot of time avoiding and procrastinating because you feel overwhelmed, only to have more and more pile up around you?

There is help, but I'm by no means an expert. So I've gathered some tools and resources to help you find ways to manage.

It takes practice, but it's well worth it! These techniques give you tangible ways to manage stress, anxiety, and fear.

- **Mindfulness**: Mindfulness is practicing being fully present in the moment, fully engaged with what you are doing and not worrying about the past or the future. Much research has shown the mental health benefits of being mindful and that it can reduce anxiety and depression. But there needs to be a balance here as well. Some people with body image concerns become overly focused on self, their bodies, or their emotions, leading to anxiety. So try not to focus on negativity but just be in the moment, keeping what's positive before you mind.

- **Reverse Bucket List**: This is a form of mindfulness that helps you become more focused on how far you've come in life and what you've accomplished. Many people have a bucket list composed of what they want to do or experience in life. This is great for goal setting. However, if you make a list of the things you are not achieving or experiencing but want to, that may add to your level of stress. It could even cause you to compare yourself to others. Try instead to make a list of the positive things that you have accomplished or experienced. Take some time each day to think about just one of those things on your list. This will help you have feelings of gratitude and appreciation for who you are, what you have accomplished, and love for the people in your life who have helped you get to where you are today.

- **Breathing techniques**: There are many methods for this form of mindfulness. When stressors arise or you feel overwhelmed by racing thoughts, simply switch to taking deep mindful breaths and count or say to yourself with each inhalation, "calmness in," and with each exhalation, "anxiety out." Or you could simply count to five backwards with each inhalation and five again with each exhalation. You can use your mind in this way to simply remove your attention from the thought that is causing stress and anxiety. There are many breathing techniques out there and you can just do an internet search and see which one speaks to you most.

- **Other tools**: If you have overwhelming stress or anxiety that is disrupting your life and the life of your family, there are therapies designed to give you tools to manage stress and your perception of stress. Again, stress is a part of our fast-paced society. So do what you can to eliminate as many stressors as you can, or their severity, and learn how to manage the stress you have no control over. Here are just two of many therapies that can give you tools and techniques that can further help with overwhelming anxiety and stress.

  1. CBT (Cognitive Behavior Therapy): CBT is an evidence-based talk therapy that helps individuals learn practical tools and techniques to reframe their thinking processes that may be distorted and cultivate positive thinking patterns (tools) that help to improve a variety

of mental health conditions like anxiety, depression, and alcohol and drug abuse.

2. DBT (Dialectical Behavior Therapy): DBT is a more specific type of CBT that helps people struggling with stronger emotional reactions. DBT teaches not only skills you would learn in CBT but also teaches skills that help them to learn what triggers their strong negative emotions and recognize their own impulsive or harmful actions.

- **Prayer**: Prayer is another wonderful mindfulness tool for those who believe in a higher power. Find a quiet place and just talk to this power like you would to a friend. Leave your problems with Him, celebrate your accomplishments with Him, and thank Him for your blessings. This can be very helpful.

SUMMARY

Stress is a reality in our fast-paced, problem-filled world. We were designed to manage short-term stress but, unfortunately, in our world stress seems to never go away. Try to find ways to reframe your way of perceiving stressful situations and learn tools to help you manage stress on a daily basis. Set aside fifteen minutes a day to practice down time, using breathing techniques or other mindfulness practices, with no outside distractions. You will quickly come to see how this helps you in the long run.

CHAPTER 5
SLEEP

— ❧ —

On average, we spend about a third of our life sleeping. An adult typically needs seven to eight hours of sleep a night. Teens usually need a bit more. But why is it that sleep is one of the first things we tend to put by the wayside when life gets hectic? Some people, often teens and young adults, just don't want to miss out on life. Others are just trying to get all their responsibilities taken care of for the day. Still others, like me, get caught up in the quiet of the night when everyone else in the house is asleep. Many of you moms know what I'm talking about. In my house, even the dog is asleep. Yes, even she instinctively knows when it's bedtime!

Sleep is so important to our well-being because that is when our body restores itself, balances out hormones, lowers stress, and regulates metabolism. Lack of that restoration can affect our mental health, hormones, and immune system. According to the CDC, "adults who were short sleepers (less than seven hours per twenty-four-hour period) were more likely to report ten chronic health conditions compared to those who got enough sleep (seven or more hours per twenty-four-hour period)." *www.cdc.gov/sleep/data_statistics.html.* This is why optimal sleep is one of the seven pillars of well-being.

WHAT HAPPENS WHEN YOU SLEEP?

Sometimes called a master clock, the body's circadian cycle is influenced mostly by light. But other environmental cues such as temperature, exercise, and social activity play a role as well. The circadian cycle produces melatonin, a hormone that signals it's time to sleep as night falls and continues being produced throughout the night to promote sleep. This plays an important role in other body systems that promote our well-being. Consider what else is going on with the body as you sleep:

- **Restoration**: The body restores itself by repairing muscle and regenerating tissue.

- **Hormones**:
  1. Appetite hormones balance out with a good night's sleep, and the digestive system slows down. With a poor nights' sleep, ghrelin and leptin are disrupted, leaving you hungrier during the day.
  2. It is thought that a good night's sleep may protect against insulin resistance and provide overall better glucose regulation.
  3. Growth hormone is released from the pituitary gland, which helps the body's processes of growth and repair.

4. Cortisol, often called the stress hormone, is regulated with a good night's sleep, which helps you feel calm and signals appropriate appetite levels when you wake up. With a bad night's sleep, cortisol (stress hormone) levels are increased during the day, leaving you feeling more stressed and less able to handle difficult situations with a calm mind.

- **The brain**: Toxins are removed and the brain declutters and reorganizes itself, getting rid of unneeded information.

- **Emotional balance**: Overreaction is more apt to occur with sleep deprivation. Decision making becomes harder, which in turn causes more stress.

- **Improved immune response**: The body releases the appropriate amount of cytokine immune proteins that help your body to lower inflammation and fight infections. This is why it's important to get plenty of sleep when you are starting to feel sick or stressed.

WHAT ARE WAYS TO IMPROVE YOUR SLEEP?

- Try to stick to a regular schedule of waking up and going to sleep each night. Usually 10 pm is optimal for turning out the lights.

- Aim for seven to nine hours of sleep nightly.

- At least two hours before going to bed, avoid bright screens or use blue blocker glasses to cut down on the blue light that encourages wakefulness. Melatonin production, that hormone needed for sleep, is influenced by light. Darkness signals the body, via this hormone, to prepare for sleep.

- Make sure the temperature in your bedroom is cool.

- Avoid eating two hours before bedtime for a number of reasons. One reason is that when the body is busy digesting food, it doesn't want to sleep. Another reason is that if you have difficulties with GERD or reflux (otherwise known as heartburn), and you lay down with food in your stomach, you are encouraging the acid in your stomach to come up.

- Avoid alcohol three to four hours before bed. Alcohol influences sleep even though you may feel relaxed. Studies have shown that alcohol will make you take longer to fall asleep and disrupt your normal sleep patterns throughout the night because of the way the body metabolizes alcohol.

- Remove or cover up all sources of lighting in your bedroom. Consider even the smallest lights from a smoke detector or clock. Get room-darkening curtains or shades to keep the artificial outside lights out. Lights affect the production of melatonin, signaling wakefulness.

- Choose relaxing activities before bedtime to help your body wind down. Some ideas for relaxation could be to read a relaxing book, take a nice warm bath with bath-salts infused with lavender essential oil, or do some stretching exercises.

- Try to get sun early in the day to reinforce natural circadian cues.

- Get some exercise or physical activity during the day. Exercise encourages sleep (but not before bed because it signals wakefulness).

- Consider caffeine; everyone is different in this regard. For instance, I'm very sensitive to caffeine and can't have any after lunch or my sleep is greatly affected. On the other hand, my husband drinks caffeine well until the evening and sleeps like a baby.

- Consider your diet as well. Recently I discovered that certain foods affect my sleep. Coconut aminos, xanthan gum, and other additives in processed foods cause me to toss and turn and wake up often. When I started eating healthier, my sleep improved.

- If you have dust mite allergies, consider encasing your pillowcases and mattress in allergy covers so you can breathe better at night.

When you are having a hard time falling asleep, change the thought pattern from "I can't sleep" to "I'll fall asleep when my body is ready." Another trick that helps me when my mind is in a vortex of thoughts is to stop and slowly count backwards from ten to one. It works because it puts the brakes on what your mind might be consumed with because your brain cannot concentrate on two things at once. Counting backwards can take concentration and be monotonous at the same time which will eventually lull the brain to sleep. Other options could be to count backwards from 100 or 300. Repeat over and over if you need to.

SUMMARY

As you can see, sleep is very important to health, and there are many factors involved in getting a good night's sleep. Try these suggestions and before you know it, you will be sleeping like a baby!

CHAPTER 6
SAFE MOVEMENT

—— ❦ ——

Safe movement! Why didn't I say "exercise"? Because exercise if not done correctly can be detrimental to well-being, and because we are all at a different place. Some struggle just to walk down their driveway while others run marathon after marathon. But one fact remains: movement done in a safe way is beneficial to health.

This chapter is where we learn to set goals. Think about having fun; exercise doesn't have to be boring. You can spend a few minutes a day putting on some music and dancing if you want. Now, don't get too crazy, I'm calling it safe movement for a reason—ha-ha! We want to improve our well-being, so the point is to find something enjoyable that you'd be more willing to stick with.

Where are you at? If you have had very little movement in your life, set a goal to do a little each day and then increase it as it becomes easier for you. If movement on a regular basis is something you are accustomed to, set a goal to move regularly or increase the amount but don't do more than is safe for your body.

What if you are a runner, a weightlifter, or an athlete of some sort? Consider whether you may be doing too much. Hear me out. Are you setting up time for recovery? In addition, more is not necessarily better. Are you exercising harder because you just seem to be losing ground with all that you have gained athletically? Could it be that you are losing ground because you are overtraining? Overtraining syndrome is real, and some of the symptoms are fatigue, loss of appetite, poor sleep, chronic joint and muscle pain, lack of motivation, moodiness, and elevated heart rate or blood pressure. What is going on in overtraining? There are several mechanisms in the body that can be affected, but let's just take cortisol, for instance. As we saw earlier, cortisol is a stress hormone that, along with other stress hormones, increases as you exercise. In moderation, normal levels keep us going, and in a fight-or-flight situation cortisol will keep you alive. However, if high levels are released on a regular basis that fight-or-flight reaction stays on and can disrupt almost all of your body's processes. The body needs regular days of rest so it can repair and strengthen. If you are not letting that happen, then the body starts to wear out. Here is a great article that explains more about what happens when you overexercise and what steps you can take to find the right balance: *www.chriskresser.com/why-you-may-need-to-exercise-less*

These are some good ways of getting in more healthy movement:

- Take the stairs instead of the elevator.

- Park your car further out in the parking lot.

- Find a fun YouTube workout you would like to do.

- Put on some good dancing music and dance while doing some household chores.

- Make a goal to walk a certain distance each day. Then push it a little further if it feels safe for you.

- Get a good app that will count your steps each day. Set a goal and increase it when you can.

The bottom line is to get up and move but do it in a safe and efficient way. Check out my website, www.functional-healthbasics.com, for my free Healthy Movement Challenge Guide. You will find more fun movement ideas in it.

SUMMARY

Healthy movement is essential to health and well-being. Try to find ways every day to get moving in a healthy and safe way. Have fun with it!

Speaking of "fun," the next chapter will help you learn why fun is a pillar of health all on its own and how important it is.

CHAPTER 7

FUN!

— ❧ —

Have some fun and laugh! Admittedly, I get too caught up in the busyness of managing life and forget to have fun. Sometimes we just need to schedule time for fun. Have you ever watched children laugh and play with no cares in the world? Don't you just love the innocence? How many times have you said, "I just wish I was a kid again with no worries"? Sadly, in today's world more and more kids are faced with adult struggles and anxieties. Look at the ability of children to go out and play and momentarily forget their woes, though. We can learn from them.

Have you heard the saying, "Laughter is the best medicine"? There is a reason for that. Studies have shown that laughter can produce a higher pain tolerance, boost immunity, lower stress hormones, relax your muscles, stop distressing emotions, and can draw others closer to us. Here's a great article from the Mayo Clinic on laughter: *www.mayoclinic.org/healthy-lifestyle/ stress-management/in-depth/stress-relief/art-20044456.*

SETTING A GOAL TO HAVE MORE FUN

- Every day, find little ways to have fun and laugh. Watch a comedy, play with a pet, read some comics, or watch some funny short clips on YouTube or TikTok.

- Weekly, on a small scale, play a game with friends and family.

- Monthly, get out and go somewhere and play. Play is whatever you want it to be. Get a group together to play basketball, go karting, go swimming, or just be with friends in general.

- Once a year go away on a vacation or take a staycation—not a TVcation. Each day get out of the house and go somewhere fun, even if just for a weekend.

- Finding ways to get out in nature can be very relaxing. Go for a hike, sit by a body of water, or have a picnic with some friends and family. Try camping as a family. Even if you don't camp, there are many options for renting stationary RVs, cabins, or other types of homes surrounded by nature.

- Check out websites and apps like Trip Advisor for ideas close by or far away.

• Google "good family getaways _____." You can fill in the blank with a destination of your choice or "near me," or "for families" or "for couples." The sky is the limit for what you can search for. Do you like sports, nature, wine, concerts, museums, or specific attractions? Use whatever your interest is for your search. Have fun with it!

SUMMARY

Life can get monotonous and busy. Take time out for having some good, balanced fun and see that you will be able to handle stress better and experience more well-being. And when you return to work, you may actually perform better. Make sure you don't play too hard, though, because that can backfire!

CHAPTER 8
AWARENESS AND APPRECIATION OF LIFE

———————————— ❧ ————————————

What is this and why is it a pillar of health and wellness? Let's face it: modern day life can move along at a crazy-fast pace. We tend to live in our own little bubbles, trying not to let obligations, work, and chronic health problems (if we have them) run us over. Sometimes, though, that's just what happens. So taking time out of our day to really think about things and appreciate the amazing joys of life all around us helps us keep on going by helping us reset. This can bring us a measure of happiness despite the chaos of our modern-day lifestyle. For instance, have you ever seen a dog dance because of pure happiness from getting a much beloved treat? My dog does that! What a happy feeling that gives my family. How about otters playing or flowers blooming? There are millions of creatures and living things to think about and enjoy. Not to mention a whole universe so vast we could never understand it all! Are you stuck inside because of winter or other reasons? Go to YouTube and look up Dog TV or Cat TV.

Try nature and see what comes up. Many people view these animal antics as something created by a higher being, that is far superior to us, for our enjoyment. If so, take the time daily to really think about why. Even if you don't believe in a God or a creator, you can still ponder about the design and joy of what you see. Why is this important? Because it lowers stress hormones, which in turn allows the body to heal and perform at its best.

WAYS TO INCREASE APPRECIATION FOR LIFE

- **Read or listen to something inspirational, spiritual, or grounding daily**: If you have a holy book, for Christians that would be the Bible, read or listen to a portion of it each day. If not, then find a book of inspirational quotes to think about daily.

- **Watch and ponder over life**: Watch your pet if you have one or just look out your window and observe the many life forms. Use a telescope when pondering the stars or YouTube when you are stuck inside or when you want to enjoy life beyond your own backdoor. Pick just one life form a day and spend five minutes observing it. (That's it! Just five minutes, or more if you have the time.) Think about how and why it does what it does. Be amused if it does something funny. Note simply how sweet or cute it is (if it is). Take note of these thoughts throughout the day.

- **Spend at least one hour a week outside**: Go for a walk in the park or set up a chair in a nature preserve. While you are using some of your stress reducing tools like breathing exercises or mindfulness to help you achieve calmness quickly, mindfully observe nature and all its beauty.

- **Pray**: If you are a religious person, take the time daily, several times in fact, to talk to God. It can be very grounding and stress relieving knowing that He has a plan.

SUMMARY

Life is very complex and interesting. Taking the time to observe it and appreciate the marvelous design and vastness all around us can bring us a measure of calmness and a feeling of inner well-being.

CHAPTER 9
BASICS OF SUPPLEMENTS

———————— ❧ ————————

Supplements, supplements, supplements—they're everywhere! How do I choose a good one? Which brand should I choose? Those are questions you may be asking. In these next three chapters, I will discuss why you may want to consider supplementing and I will give you some ideas of what to specifically look for in supplements to make sure you get a good quality one. I will also discuss specific basic supplements that support the immune system and others that replace nutrients that you may be lacking.

Perhaps you've heard some experts say that all you need to do is to eat a healthy diet to get all the nutrients you need and that supplements are not necessary. On the other hand, maybe you have heard the other side of the spectrum where some experts have a huge list of supplements they feel everyone should take. So who do you believe?

Think back to all you have learned in this guide. You learned the basics and yet I hope you got a clear picture of the many reasons we could be lacking in certain nutrients. So in this chapter I'm going to talk about the areas of biggest concern and why targeting certain areas of vitamin and mineral depletions will be the best approach possible.

First, there is no "one size fits all." We are all different and a multivitamin typically will not get you what you need. Second, consider what your symptoms, diagnoses, diet, and lifestyle are like. For instance, someone with Crohn's, celiac, or other gut issues will not absorb nutrients the way that the gut was meant to. Someone who eats a vegan diet may not be getting enough vitamin B-12. Another example is vitamin D. Most people living above a certain latitude are deficient in vitamin D and on top of that, the darker the skin, the more deficient. I discovered, years ago, that I felt better in the summertime when the kids and I were outside soaking up the sun. Little did I know that my vitamin D was extremely deficient in the winters, which set me up for seasonal depression and one sickness after another every single year. Now that I'm supplementing, I sail through winters with absolutely no depression, as well as no colds or flu for the last five years. Much can be said about that nutrient alone.

THE BASICS OF WHAT TO LOOK FOR IN SUPPLEMENTS

Ingredients matter. Look for a very limited amount of inactive ingredients. Generally, capsules are the best options. Avoid supplements with fillers and look for a statement that it is free from gluten, dairy, and many other common allergens.

Another consideration is where to get your supplements from. As much as I don't like the inconvenience sometimes involved with good sources for supplements, it's a valid concern. Be aware of buying on Amazon. There have been many reports of knockoffs slipping into the supply at the world's largest online retailer. Buying direct from the manufacturer, your doctor, or another reputable source are better options than Amazon. I used to buy on Amazon all the time, but I started to notice some quality issues with certain supplements I was buying. So now, despite how much of a pain it is, I buy most of my supplements from reputable sources. This prevents me from getting knockoffs that may not even contain the nutrient I am buying them for or, worse, getting a supplement that may be tainted with potentially harmful ingredients.

To summarize what basics to look for:

- Limit inactive ingredients

- Capsules are better than other forms (except for liposomal liquid forms, which I get into more later)

- Buy from a reputable source, not Amazon

So let's talk a little about some of these supplements. There are numerous supplements out there and many have needed benefits while others are just money makers. Next are a few categories I feel are important: supporting the immune system and replacing nutrients that may be lacking. Both categories can also go hand in hand. Nutrients that support the immune system may also be replacing a deficiency and the supplements that may be replacing a deficiency may also support the immune system. Now, more than ever, people are wanting to find ways to support their immune system so that's my next topic on supplements.

CHAPTER 10
IMMUNE-SUPPORTING
SUPPLEMENTS

—————————— ✿ ——————————

Because of the recent pandemic, I thought that immune support should be where we start. For instance, as time has passed there have been **many** studies that have been done that show that higher vitamin D levels are linked to better outcomes with COVID-19. Other vitamins and minerals are beneficial, as well, for immune support. The top three that I'll address are vitamin D, vitamin C, and zinc.

VITAMIN D

Vitamin D is a fat-soluble vitamin we need for optimal regulation and function of the body. Many studies have shown that this vitamin helps to trigger the expression of more than two hundred health-supporting genes and that it is beneficial for various chronic conditions such as diabetes, cancer, asthma, and osteoporosis. It can help regulate the immune system and promote neuromuscular function. Getting too little may affect other hormones like cortisol and thyroid.

Vitamin D can be found in a variety of foods, although not enough to get the optimal levels needed for its healthy benefits. The best way to get vitamin D is from sun exposure. Absorption of ultraviolet rays triggers the body to make vitamin D. If you live in a climate where you are inside during the winter season, your vitamin D may not be built up to optimal levels. Also, if you do spend a lot of time outdoors but slather on sunscreen and sunblock, your body won't be able to build up the vitamin D as well. When you are able to get sun exposure, the amount of vitamin D your body will produce from daily sun exposure will depend on your skin type, skin color, your burn threshold, how much skin you expose, and the cloud cover. Everyone is different so that's where vitamin D supplementation comes in. How much should you take and where should you get it?

This is where the controversy arises. The recommended daily amount by the IOM (Institute of Medicine) is 600 international units (IU) and recommended serum (blood) levels of 20 ng/ml. This is the amount that was determined years ago to prevent severe deficiency that leads to rickets, a rare condition that disturbs normal bone growth in children leading to skeletal deformities and growth delays. However, there has been a vast amount of current scientific research and data that shows that number is way too low. Many scientists and doctors are recommending that serum levels be between 40 and 60 ng/ml. The Institute for Functional Medicine (IFM) advises between 50 and 80 ng/ml. So the best target should be around 50 and 60 ng/ml.

There are cautions when taking vitamin D. First, if you have parathyroid or liver problems, talk with your doctor because of some potential hazards with vitamin D intake with those conditions. Second, if you don't know your blood serum levels, it is recommended that you take no more than 2,000 IU a day. Monitoring your blood levels is the safest way to assure that you are taking appropriate amounts. Although extremely rare, vitamin D can bioaccumulate, and toxicity can occur, leading to hypercalcemia, frequent kidney problems, excessive urination, loss of appetite, nausea, and vomiting. Generally, this toxicity level doesn't happen until you reach serum levels of 100 ng/ml. The best plan for increasing your vitamin D levels is to talk to your doctor about getting lab work done to show where your levels are and to continue monitoring so that your levels don't get too high. Two other options are www.grassrootshealth.net where you can have a kit sent to you for testing. Once your test results come back, they also have a chart for knowing how much vitamin D to take to get to optimal levels. The other option is ordering your own lab work if you are in a state where it is legal. It may even cheaper than most labs if you don't have insurance or if you have a very high deductible. On my website you will find a good lab and a link to it, or you can do an internet search to find your own lab.

Some other helpful information is to make sure that you take vitamin D3 (vitamin D2 is synthetic and not as efficient at increasing blood levels). Take vitamin D3 with vitamin K2 because they work together for optimal efficiency and bone strengthening. Also make sure that your magnesium levels are good so that you can absorb calcium effectively. Vitamin D is fat soluble so take it with some dietary fat to promote absorption. I personally like the liquid form of the Thorne brand because it is mixed with dietary fat and because I have celiac disease and don't absorb nutrients as well. One other note to consider: don't wait until you are sick to start taking vitamin D! Vitamin D, at optimal levels, works best with the immune system *before* you get sick.

To learn more about vitamin D, read this excellent article on common myths that you may have heard about vitamin D: *https://www.grassrootshealth.net/project/top-10-vitamin-d-myths-whats-fact-whats-not*

ZINC

Zinc is an essential mineral that your body cannot produce on its own. So, you need to get zinc from dietary sources or supplementation. Quite a bit of research has shown that zinc is important for immune function. Zinc is also beneficial for managing inflammation and promoting good bone health. You can find zinc in every cell of your body and it is needed not only for immunity but for reproduction, growth, and thyroid function. Usually 15 to 30 mg a day is what is typically recommended. Maybe a little more if you develop a cold or other infection. Too much can lead to copper deficiency, so keep that in mind. Good dietary sources of zinc are found in meat, legumes, nuts, and eggs.

VITAMIN C

Most likely you have heard of taking vitamin C when you have a cold. That's because it is a beneficial antioxidant. However, vitamin C is also beneficial for helping with stress and increasing energy levels. It also affects how we express our DNA and genetic activity.

The problem with vitamin C is that the body doesn't make it, so it only stores a little at a time. That means it is essential to get what we can from dietary sources as well as supplementation. The best sources of dietary vitamin C are fruits and vegetables, particularly citrus fruits, strawberries, tomatoes, and cruciferous vegetables like broccoli, cauliflower, cabbage, and brussels sprouts. For supplementation, there are four types of vitamin C: ascorbic acid, ester C (or calcium ascorbate), vitamin C with bioflavonoids, and liposomal vitamin C. It's important that you understand the differences among them because then you can choose one that will work optimally with your body and your needs while also saving you money.

- **Ascorbic acid** is probably the most common form of vitamin C that you will find. The problem with this form is that it is acidic and will irritate sensitive digestive systems.

- **Calcium ascorbate or Ester C** is less acidic than ascorbic acid and is better absorbed by the body. Not only is this a better option for individuals who have digestive issues, some doctors and researchers feel that this is a good option for allergy sufferers because this form reduces the histamine levels in the body.

- **Vitamin C with bioflavonoids** allows the body to use the vitamin C more effectively because the bioflavonoids enhance the bioavailability of the vitamin C in the body. However, check to see that the actual form of the vitamin C is calcium ascorbate and not ascorbic acid for even better protection for the digestive system.

- **Liposomal vitamin C** is the best of the best. Especially if you have digestive issues. Found in liquid form, liposomal vitamin C can be absorbed into cells, thus protecting the digestive system from irritation and vitamin breakdown. Many supplements are available in liposomal form. With liposomal supplements, nutrients are encapsulated into liposomes, which are tiny nano-sized fat particles that keep the nutrient from being broken down in the digestive system. Instead, because they are so small, they can be easily absorbed into the cells of the body. Here is a great liposomal vitamin C: *https://www.quicksilverscientific.com/all-products/liposomal-vitamin-c/*.

- **IV vitamin C** is a fifth form of vitamin C that I just wanted you to be aware of. It is a very high-dose option that is easily usable by the body and totally avoids any gastrointestinal upset. But, for obvious reasons this is not a form that you can manage yourself. Many functional medicine practitioners as well as other health care professionals offer this form.

The RDA (recommended daily allowance) of vitamin C is 75 mg per day for adult women and 90 mg per day for adult men and the recommended "tolerable upper intake level" was set at 2000 mg per day in the USA and Canada. Two-thousand mg per day is the "upper tolerable limit" according to the Food and Nutrition Board (FNB) at the Institute of Medicine (IOM); it's the maximum amount at which, they feel, vitamin C will be unlikely to cause adverse health effects. That said, vitamin C toxicity from mega doses is virtually unheard of. Those with kidney failure should use caution and speak to their doctor about mega dose vitamin C.

CHAPTER 11
REPLACEMENT NUTRIENTS

— ❧ —

Now that we have covered a few supplements that will help your immune system and offer other benefits, let's look next at nutrients many people are deficient in.

MAGNESIUM

Magnesium is available in many foods like greens (spinach, kale, and Swiss chard), nuts and seeds (pumpkin seeds, cashews, almonds, and flax seed), as well as cooked beans. Unfortunately, many people don't get enough in their diet because they eat too many processed foods, which strip the food of its magnesium.

Magnesium is essential for over three hundred processes in our body and helps with hormone regulation. Low levels of magnesium are linked to insulin resistance, weight gain, type-2 diabetes, and even restless leg syndrome. Certain forms such as magnesium L-threonate have been proven in studies to cross over the blood brain barrier and are useful for stress management, relaxation, and sleep. Magnesium glycinate is known to be easier on the stomach, doesn't cause diarrhea in most people, and is easier to absorb. The RDA of magnesium is 400 mg per day for men and 310 mg per day for women. If you are severely lacking in magnesium, your healthcare provider can recommend a dose that's right for you.

Some symptoms of magnesium deficiency:

- Muscle cramping
- Frequent headaches or migraines
- Anxiety and depression
- PMS
- Low energy
- Trouble sleeping
- Restless leg syndrome

B VITAMINS

B vitamins are beneficial for healthy metabolism, nerve function, the formation of red blood cells, and DNA production. You can find plenty of dietary sources of B vitamins in meat, eggs, legumes, seeds, and leafy greens. B12 is highest in meats. There are several reasons for B12 deficiency. For instance, an individual who primarily eats a vegetarian or vegan diet may be lacking in B12 because of avoiding B12-containing meats. For others, they may have a methylation impairment like the MTHFR gene mutation that impairs the way the body metabolizes and converts dietary nutrients into usable forms in the body. Diet and high levels of stress can also deplete our levels of B vitamins.

Some symptoms of vitamin B deficiencies are fatigue, weakness, heart palpitations, brain fog, diarrhea, constipation, anemia, and tingling in the hands and feet. B12, B6, and folate deficiencies can be linked to depression, anxiety, and obsessive-compulsive disorder (OCD). In fact, many practitioners have begun to treat OCD with the B vitamin inositol.

The best way to get your Bs are through diet as well as learning strategies to manage your stress so your body doesn't deplete your B vitamins. If you suspect you have methylation problems, talk with a functional medicine practitioner to verify or go to my website, www.functionalhealthbasics.com, for a link to a lab where you can order your own test. If you do have the MTHFR mutation, supplement with B-complex vitamins that contain methylated B vitamins. B vitamins are also available in the liposomal form which, as we went over earlier, encapsulates the vitamins in small nanoparticles for better transport throughout the body. If you are a vegan or vegetarian, consider getting your B12 levels drawn to see if you are getting enough B12 in your diet. If you are not getting enough then consider eating more B12-rich foods like sunflower seeds, kidney and lima beans, and brewer's and torula yeast. Your doctor may prescribe vitamin B12 shots or supplements for you to take.

PROBIOTICS

Our intestines are filled with bacteria, fungi, and other microorganisms. This is called the gut microbiome. Our bodies were designed to have a proper balance of these microorganisms for a healthy body. When the microbiome is out of balance then everything about our health can be affected. It can affect our stress response, carbohydrate digestion, fat storage, and immune system health. It can also affect our mental health, bring on acid reflux, and cause constipation or diarrhea.

We tend to become unbalanced because of genetics, a poor diet, antibiotics, and other medications. Considering how much our gut microbiome affects much of our health, it's wise to take probiotics into consideration when we are dealing with chronic health problems. Many individuals have reported a decline in many of their symptoms with the use of probiotics.

Symptoms vary:

- Bloating, diarrhea, constipation, and gas

- Signs and symptoms of body-wide inflammation such as fatigue, brain fog, depression, anxiety, insomnia, and hormone imbalances

- Autoimmunity

- Signs of poor nutrient absorption such as dry brittle hair and dry skin, as well as fatigue.

When choosing probiotics what are the best options for supplementing? There are endless options out there to choose from and many are just not worth the money. On top of that every person is different as to how they will tolerate certain formulations because no two people are balanced the same. I suggest looking for a good high-quality probiotic from reputable sources such as Thorne. You can order from them on a sub-scription basis and get a discount as well as free shipping. I personally have found that a soil based (SBO) probiotic works great for me. Amy Meyers, MD, is a well-known functional medicine provider who has a good soil-based probiotic. Another way to get good probiotics is eating a diet full of plenty of fermented foods, such as sauerkraut, yogurt (there are dairy free options available), and apple cider vinegar.

When taking probiotics, making sure that you get good prebiotics is important. Prebiotics are healthy fibers from a variety of fruits and vegetables that the good bacteria in your body feed on to remain stable. Good sources of prebiotics are root vegetables, bananas, apples, berries, whole grains, seeds, and legumes. Fermented foods are also good because they include prebiotics with the probiotics.

A caution about prebiotics and probiotics is that people with digestive problems such as SIBO, IBS, or FODMAP intolerance need to use caution and see a functional medicine practitioner to address those problems first. Soil-based probiotics tend to be a probiotic of choice with these conditions.

SECTION 2 SUMMARY: SUPPLEMENTS

Supplements are not necessarily for everyone, and each person is unique. So when considering supplements, consider your personal needs. Does your bloodwork show any deficiencies? Do you have certain nutrients lacking in your diet? How much sun do you get? Are you trying to build up your immune system or treat certain illnesses? These are personal things to consider that will be unique to you. And remember, if you decide to take supplements, make sure you are buying good quality ones from reputable sources.

INFLAMMATION

Functional Medicine vs Conventional Medicine for Specific Conditions

⎯⎯⎯⎯⎯⎯⎯ 🌿 ⎯⎯⎯⎯⎯⎯⎯

In the following chapters, I'm going to simply list various chronic conditions or wellness obstacles that people have and compare the different approaches of conventional and functional medicine. If you have a condition not listed here, try doing an internet search for your condition and add the words "functional medicine" to it. This is how you can continue to learn about how functional medicine can be useful in your health recovery.

Because chronic inflammation is at the root of many disease processes, I start with that in this chapter. As we discuss other chronic conditions in the following chapters you will come to see that inflammation has a common root in many of them.

WHAT IS INFLAMMATION?

Inflammation is when the body's immune system sends out inflammatory cells to do what is needed to heal damaged tissue or get rid of a pathogen, like a bacteria or virus. So inflammation is a good thing when it is healing the body from sudden injuries or infections. But when the body is constantly inflamed, it can lead to autoimmune diseases, poor healing, and other illnesses such as cancer. In fact, many researchers feel that inflammation is at the root of most chronic disease, including many mental health conditions.

WHAT CAUSES CHRONIC INFLAMMATION?

- **Chronic infections**: Chronic infections are infections that the immune system hasn't been able to eradicate. Lyme disease and Epstein-Barr virus are just two examples of pathogens the body isn't properly getting rid of. In recent years, another example is the COVID-19 virus that has left people with what is called long COVID or post-COVID syndrome.

- **Nutritional deficiencies**: Nutritional deficiencies, such as Vitamin D, Vitamin B12, magnesium, etc., have been associated with inflammation. Not that they are the direct cause but adequate levels are needed for the immune system to function properly.

- **Toxins**: Toxins are substances produced naturally, or they can be man-made. The body's immune system, if properly nourished, is designed to take care of the occasional exposure to toxins. However, in our world today, we are constantly exposed. Each one of us has a tolerance level.

Let's just call that tolerance level a bucket and note that some buckets are bigger than others. What that means is that some people with bigger buckets can tolerate a large amount of toxic exposure and not have any ill effects. Then there are some of us who, for various reasons, have smaller buckets. So when individuals are chronically exposed to toxins, whether from chemicals in personal care products, pollution, mold exposure, too much sugar, or a combination of chemicals, their bucket overflows. When the bucket overflows, chronic, ongoing inflammation occurs. Another illustration is the canary in a mine, which we used as metaphor earlier. Miners knew that when the canary died it was time to leave the mine because the toxins were too high. The canary had a small bucket! Consider the size of your bucket. How are you managing the toxins in your environment? You can read more about toxins in chapter 3.

- **Stress**: Stress can cause chronic inflammation. Our bodies were designed to manage acute stressful situations by activating the nerves and hormones, like cortisol, for instance. This response is called the "fight or flight" reaction. If something scares you, your body immediately goes into action to respond for your own survival. This response affects your nerves, hormones, heart, insulin levels, and gut. This is a great response if you were to cross paths with a bear when you are hiking in the woods!

  The problem with chronic, ongoing stress, whether physical or mental, is that the body doesn't know the difference between life-threatening and benign stress. So the body reacts in the same way to everyday modern stressors, causing our hormones like cortisol, adrenalin, and glucagon to be constantly activated, which leads to chronic inflammation. (See chapter 4 for stress-management tools.) We cannot get rid of stress entirely, but we can learn how to find ways to lower stress by living a simpler life or find ways to manage or balance out the stress we have no control over.

- **Variety of foods**: Foods that are inflammatory to many people are gluten, dairy, sugar, modern grains, refined and processed carbs such as bread and pastries, sugar-sweetened beverages, excessive alcohol, processed foods, and artificially unhealthy fats and oils. Foods you may be sensitive or allergic to will also be inflammatory. Doing an investigative elimination diet can help you find the foods that trigger inflammation in your body.

SYMPTOMS OF CHRONIC INFLAMMATION

- Pain
- Brain fog
- Joint pain
- Fatigue
- Lack of attention
- Headaches
- Sleep disruption

MANAGING INFLAMMATION

We can lower the inflammation in our bodies by addressing the areas that may be contributing to it in the first place. The

3 Rs come into play here. **Remove** anything that may be causing our body harm. **Replace** what may be missing for your body to function optimally, and **Repair** what may be broken (like a leaky gut, for instance). This is where a functional medicine doctor or practitioner can come in handy by being a detective and ordering tests as indicated. Or a health coach can be of use in helping you to be your own detective by making appropriate suggestions.

CHAPTER 13
WEIGHT LOSS

—— ❧ ——

Is your main goal to lose weight? Let's say you feel just fine but you want to shed a few pounds. Then use this chapter to set your goals. A word of caution, though: weight loss involves more than calories in and out. High stress levels can impede weight loss because the hormones that support the fight-or-flight response to stress may actually cause weight gain. Environmental toxins called endocrine disruptors can also wreak havoc on the endocrine (hormone) system, preventing weight loss. Lack of good quality sleep and inflammatory foods can also prevent weight loss. Using the pillars in this book—like stress, fun, sleep, and food, for instance—can be very beneficial in helping you reach your goals. Something else to consider is age. If you are a female, are you closing in on menopause? Yes, those hormone changes can cause weight gain. Speak with your doctor about bioidentical hormone replacement therapy. Here is what my functional medicine doctor, who used to be a gynecologist, has to say about it on her blog:

https://vitalityrenewal.org/how-conventional-medicine-got-hormone-replacement-all-wrong/. This can make a huge difference! It did for me!

I've mentioned elimination diets and the paleo diet in the chapter on food; however, in this chapter we are going to get further in depth as to how it relates to weight loss and the differences between these diets. Why do people report feeling great on paleo, keto, and vegan diets? That's because, generally, they are eating more fruits and vegetables as well as avoiding the SAD American Diet (SAD). Past dietary philosophies, such as low-calorie diets or low-fat diets, have proven to be more detrimental to weight loss. I spent all my teen and early adult life trying diets that incorporate these philosophies only to gain more and more weight. For instance, low-calorie diets send the body into a fat-retention mode and encourage it to burn muscle for energy, leading to even more weight gain as time goes on. Low-fat diets are detrimental because our bodies were designed to need healthy fats to survive. In fact, when I started adding healthy fats to my diet I started to lose weight. Coming from years of the "you can't lose weight by eating fatty foods" mentality, the weight loss took me by surprise. I was saying to myself, "Can this really be so?" There is a lot that can be said about this and if you want to know more, here is a great article that explains why low-fat diets are actually bad for you: www. drwillcole.com/functional-medicine/low-fat-diets-are-no-good. But for now let's focus on some of the better dietary choices out there.

BETTER DIETARY CHOICES

- **Paleo**: The "pros" include plenty of whole foods, fiber, and nutrients. It utilizes almost all the food groups, except for grains and dairy, which can be inflammatory for many. Those with autoimmune diseases tend to do well on this type of diet. A "con" is that avoiding grains may be challenging for some.

- **Keto**: The closest diet to paleo, one that's all the rave lately, is the ketogenic diet. It's similar because the main food groups are meats and some vegetables. However, fruits, and other carbs are very low if at all. Many find this diet good for quick weight loss yet struggle to sustain eating this way for the long term and quickly revert to poor eating habits.

    Pros: Weight loss can be quick and some experts endorse it for type-2 diabetes. *Cons:* Keto eliminates healthy food groups that are high in nutrients, it can be excessively high in saturated fat, it contains some inflammatory foods like dairy, there is a potential for low fiber intake, and the diet is hard to maintain for a long period of time.

- **Vegan**: Pros: high in fiber, vegetables, and nutrients. Cons: some may find it difficult to get enough protein, and it may involve foods that are inflammatory to some people such as grains. Also, vegans and vegetarians may need vitamin B12 and iron due to avoiding meats.

A big caution for all of these diets and any other diet: watch out for foods that are processed and marketed for these diets (diet bars, baked goods, and meatless meats) because they have the potential to be high in sugar and other added processed ingredients that can be inflammatory to the body and actually work against your goals. The best approach is to eat as much whole foods as possible. Cut out the sugar and save that paleo, keto, or vegan cookie for a special occasion.

Resource articles for weight loss:

www.amymyersmd.com/article/weight-loss-functional-medicine
www.drhyman.com/blog/2017/08/10/cant-lose-weight

CHAPTER 14
GASTROESOPHAGEAL REFLUX DISEASE (GERD)

—— ❧ ——

As we saw, GERD stands for gastroesophageal reflux disease. It's basically a chronic form of gastric reflux because the symptoms of reflux happen more than twice a week on a regular basis. Symptoms are heartburn, regurgitation of the stomach contents, chest pain, chronic cough, and difficulty swallowing. Some of the symptoms may even be confused with asthma. What happens when a person has gastric reflux is that the acid in the stomach backs up into the esophagus (the tube from the mouth to the stomach), which can cause a burning sensation or warming sensation in the chest. That's why some people call it heartburn. Sometimes the gastric contents come all the way up into the mouth. I remember the first time this happened to me. I was pregnant, and in the middle of the night, bam! It woke me out of a deep sleep. It can be very uncomfortable at the very least, but left untreated, the esophagus can become eroded, leading to scarring, constriction, ulcers, and even cancer of the esophagus.

There are many causes of gastric reflux. But the underlying causes and treatments are very different between functional medicine and conventional. Both conventional and functional medicine will look at these contributing factors:

- A large belly, either related to weight gain or pregnancy. The size of the abdomen may push up against the stomach, nudging the contents upward and weakening the valve from the stomach to the esophagus.

- Eating before bedtime.

- Eating meals that are too big.

- Foods that are known to aggravate reflux like spicy foods, chocolate, tomatoes, fried fatty foods, processed foods, alcohol, caffeine, and peppermint.

Doctors of conventional medicine believe that the gastric fluid of the stomach is too acidic and will basically treat the acid reflux with antacids or other acid blockers to lower the acid content in the stomach. Does this work? Sure it works! It seems to make sense because the acid is coming up the esophagus. But here's a question to consider: why do doctors of functional medicine have such great success with treating the opposite way by *increasing* the acid content of the stomach to treat gastric reflux? Not that this is the way they always treat gastric reflux, but if it is indicated, they will recommend betaine HCL with pepsin to increase the acid content. I was having problems with acid reflux for a while and I used this supplement, which improved my reflux greatly. Before this, I had been taking antacids from time to time, and when a flare-up occurred at night I would simply take an antacid and sleep with my head elevated to help. My son, on the other hand, actually had GERD and was treated with some pretty strong meds. After he was diagnosed with Celiac disease he started eating gluten free and avoided trigger foods. His symptoms improved so much that he was able to completely get off medications.

Practitioners of functional medicine will see gastric reflux as a symptom of an underlying problem, so they will look for a potential root cause of the gastric reflux or GERD. That's because taking acid-blocking meds or other types of medications can lead to other problems such as nutrient deficiencies. Our stomach was designed to have a high acid level in order to break down food for proper nutrient absorption.

Here are some other factors that functional practitioners look for.

- Food sensitivities (beyond the common triggers) like dairy and gluten.

- An overgrowth of bad bacteria or yeast in your stomach because of a lot of antibiotics, eating too much sugar, or other factors. The overgrowth throws off the normal balance of the stomach and can lead to acid reflux.

- H-pylori infection of the stomach.

- Low magnesium can affect the stomach's ability to move the food contents along to the upper intestines.

- Chronic stress leads to an imbalanced nervous system that will affect how the stomach processes food.

- Low acid. Many of the conditions I mentioned above are related to low stomach acid in one way or another. Stomach acid is needed for keeping the stomach healthy and the microbiome of the stomach balanced. So when the acid is low, carbs are not absorbed properly and bad bacteria and yeast feed off of them, causing gas and abdominal pressure. This in turn causes the sphincter leading up to the esophagus to relax and open, allowing the stomach contents to come up.

Examples of how a practitioner of functional medicine will treat GERD or gastric reflux are as follows:

- **Reduce** or eliminate the triggering foods, encourage weight loss and a low carb diet, look for food sensitivities, and treat any infection. Avoid ibuprofen, aspirin, and other NSAIDS that are known to be irritating to the stomach.

- **Replace** what is missing: they will look for magnesium deficiency and work to increase the acid content of the stomach by supplementing with HCL with pepsin (you won't want to do this until you have healed any ulcers you may have first). Doctors may even add probiotics if SIBO (small intestinal bacterial overgrowth) isn't an issue.

- **Repair** the esophagus and stomach by allowing it to repair itself by doing the first two previous steps to prevent further damage. They may also recommend l-glutamine, bone broth, collagen, and deglycerized licorice (DLG), which support the healing of the gut and calm gut inflammation.

Many individuals choose to take the challenge of healing of their own gut on their own. I've included the following articles from functional medicine practitioners I trust in hopes that it may be of use to you on your journey:

https://drhyman.com/blog/2013/09/26/7-steps-reverse-acid-reflux/

https://chriskresser.com/how-to-cure-gerd-without-medication/

https://www.amymyersmd.com/article/gerd/

CHAPTER 15

FIBROMYALGIA

———————— ❧ ————————

Have you been diagnosed with fibromyalgia? Are you suffering from body-wide muscular pain that just doesn't go away? Do you have difficulty concentrating, brain fog, difficulty sleeping, or just want to sleep all day? According to the Mayo Clinic, "Fibromyalgia often coexists with other conditions" (*https://www.mayoclinic.org/diseases-conditions/ fibromyalgia/symptoms-causes/syc-20354780*). Do you have some of these conditions: irritable bowel syndrome, chronic fatigue syndrome, anxiety, depression, or migraine disorders?

If you do, then my heart goes out to you because of the difficulties you are facing. Doctors of conventional medicine may be genuinely trying to help you with pain medication, sleeping pills, antidepressants, or other means. Their aim is to manage the symptoms of pain, difficulty sleeping, or depression. But why are the symptoms there in the first place? Fibromyalgia itself is a symptom of inflammation that indicates that there is an imbalance of the immune system, nervous system, or endocrine system. (See chapter 12.) The approach of a functional medicine practitioner will look for the root cause of why those systems may be imbalanced in the first place. Consider what those causes could be:

- Thyroid imbalances. The thyroid can cause widespread pain if it is not balanced properly, and thyroid disorders are commonly overlooked or not treated to the optimum degree. Because of that, I write about the thyroid further in chapter 17. There can be other hormone imbalances such as cortisol, estrogen, and progesterone. Perhaps these imbalances are related to chronic stress or age.

- Nutritional deficiencies such as magnesium, vitamins B12 and D, and glutathione. There could be a genetic component to nutritional deficiencies such as a MTHFR mutation that will disrupt proper methylating of the nutrients. If so, this prevents the body from properly detoxifying toxins. As toxins build up, the body stores them and inflammation results.

- Food sensitives and gluten intolerance.

- Chronic undiagnosed infections from parasites, bacteria, or yeast.

- Exposure to mycotoxins produced from toxic mold.

These are just some of the avenues that functional medicine will take when it comes to conditions like fibromyalgia and chronic fatigue syndrome. If you read my story, then you are aware that I too had been diagnosed with fibromyalgia and chronic fatigue syndrome earlier in my life. I am no longer plagued with these maladies. Functional medicine gave me my life back! For me, it was a combination of underlying causes. And if I don't eat right or my hormones are not at their optimal levels, then I will start to see symptoms returning.

I hope this chapter helps you see that you don't have to have a life of chronic pain and fatigue if you are willing to dig deeper and make changes. Perhaps the stress of the journey or the changes you would have to make are too overwhelming. That's alright! Each and every one of us is an individual who knows what path is best for us and our own unique circumstance.

In the next chapter, I'm going to show you the differences between how functional medicine and conventional medicine tackle anxiety and depression. These challenges may go along with fibromyalgia and chronic fatigue, so perhaps you would like to take a peek.

Here is an excellent article about fibromyalgia and another about functional medicine in general:

https://www.amymyersmd.com/article/fibromyalgia-functional -medicine/

https://chriskresser.com/why-we-get-sick-and-how-to-get-well/

CHAPTER 16
ANXIETY AND DEPRESSION

———————————— ❧ ————————————

Anxiety and depression are rampant in our society. I don't think there is anyone who doesn't know someone who struggles with it. Years back, I suffered from post-partum depression as well as seasonal depression. I remember wanting to drive my van directly into a semi-truck to get it all done and over with. At the time, the only thing that stopped me was the thought of what my babies would do without a mother. I did not know then what I know now, and I was too embarrassed to admit how bad my depression was. But looking back, I should have told my doctor just how bad it was. As for the seasonal depression, that was simply resolved by getting my vitamin D up to good therapeutic levels. (For more on vitamin D, see chapter 10.) But that is not going to be the answer for everyone. Before we get further into this discussion, I want to make it very clear that if you are on an antidepressant, do not stop taking it without the approval of a doctor. And if you are depressed, please don't hesitate to contact a doctor to help you feel better. There is a way out! You may choose a conventional approach with medication or you may choose to look deeper with a functional medicine practitioner. Either way is fine, but don't let yourself suffer. Your life is way too important. The information I am providing here is just that: information. What you will learn will help you navigate and decide for yourself if you want to explore further what the root causes of your mental health struggles are. You may even choose to use both conventional and functional medicine in your journey. My son, for instance, deals with anxiety and depression. His past choice was antidepressants for depression and anxiety but now he wants to keep taking the medications and explore what else could be going on. He is ready to eat healthier and do what else he can to feel better. With him it has been hard to even find medication that works and that doesn't leave him with terrible side effects. So, let's dive in and learn more about these two conditions.

Depression can range from feeling blue to feeling like life is not worth living. If you are depressed to the point of feeling like life is not worth living, I beg you to please see your doctor immediately! Life is worth living and you are worthy to be alive. This leads me to the conventional approach. Conventional doctors will try to help you manage symptoms with medication, therapy, exercise, and other tools like mindfulness. If you are dealing with severe depression or anxiety, it is alright to take medicine. But perhaps you don't like taking medicine. Think of it this way: it's the beginning of a journey that may help you get to the point where you can be more proactive in your decisions and understanding.

When you are facing a mental health crisis, it is in control of you—let's face it. When you start to gain some control of your life, you can then start to explore some of the root causes as to why you are suffering. As you find answers and solutions, eventually you may be able to get off medication for good. So let's explore what some of those root causes of anxiety and depression may be.

- **Imbalanced gut**. There is a saying in functional medicine: "Fire in the gut, fire in the brain," which means that if your gut, meaning the intestines, colon, or stomach, is off-balance because of bacterial imbalance, parasites, celiac, or some other cause, then inflammation occurs, which effects the brain. This is also known as the gut-brain connection. You can do a quick internet search and you will see that the "gut-brain connection" is well known within the scientific and medical community. Sadly, many doctors and psychiatrists are not aware of this connection, and if they are, it's not within the scope of how they are taught to practice medicine.

- **Adrenal and other hormonal imbalances, like the HPA axis dysfunction**. Often chronic stress will keep you in a state of panic and throw off the stress hormones such as cortisol and DHEA, which alters the neurotransmitters in the brain. Chronic inflammation can also throw off the stress hormones. Learning how to manage stress and inflammation can be of great benefit.

- **Nutritional deficiencies can be a culprit**. Vitamin D, zinc, omega-3 fatty acids, B12, magnesium, and other nutrients are linked to mood. Getting them checked and maintaining them at the right levels can make a difference. Eating a whole food diet can be beneficial as well.

The bottom line is that there are answers out there and you have good reasons to hope that you can feel better than you do now. I've included some very good articles below on the subject from experts that I highly regard in the functional medicine community.

https://drhyman.com/blog/2015/09/18/6-strategies-to-eliminate-depression/

https://chriskresser.com/functional-medicine-approach-depression/

https://chriskresser.com/functional-medicine-approach-to-anxiety/

https://grassrootsfunctionalmedicine.com/blog/functional-medicine-anxiety/

https://drbrighten.com/healing-anxiety-functional-medicine/

CHAPTER 17

THYROID CONDITIONS

D o you have a thyroid condition? Maybe it is under-active or overactive? Most people with thyroid conditions have underactive thyroids. But I'm going to list some of the symptoms of both hyper- and hypoactive thyroids and how doctors will treat the conditions.

OVERACTIVE THYROID

Let's start with a hyperactive thyroid. A hyperactive thyroid can come from an autoimmune condition called Grave's disease. When this autoimmune condition occurs, the body's immune system attacks the thyroid, causing it to produce too much T4 (thyroxine), which in turn ramps up the body's metabolism. Symptoms of too much T4 are unintended weight loss, dry brittle hair and skin, hair loss, heart palpitations or irregularity, sweating, heat intolerance, changes in the menstrual pattern, increased appetite, anxiety, irritability, and an enlarged thyroid (goiter) that appears at the base of the neck.

Complications of untreated hyperthyroid levels are increased risk of stroke, congestive heart failure, brittle bones (osteoporosis), thyroid crisis, and Grave's ophthalmopathy. Sometimes, especially with smokers, a condition associated with Grave's, ophthalmopathy, will occur that makes the eyeballs protrude beyond what is normal. My mother suffered from this for the rest of her life after the time that she was in the hospital to have her thyroid removed. I remember that she always had to tape her eyelids closed when she went to bed to protect her eyes from damage and from drying out.

What do conventional doctors do to treat hyperactive thyroids? They may prescribe anti-thyroid medications or doses of radioactive iodine. Sometimes they may even remove part or all of the thyroid. The approach functional medicine practitioners take to an overactive thyroid is similar to the one they take to an underactive thyroid. To read more about Grave's disease I included a link at the end of this chapter. In the meantime, let's dive into underactive thyroids.

UNDERACTIVE THYROID

An underactive thyroid (hypothyroidism) fails to produce enough thyroid hormones and leads to some similar symptoms of an overactive thyroid, but mostly the symptoms are the opposite of an overactive thyroid. Underactive thyroid conditions are mostly autoimmune related. This is called Hashimoto's thyroiditis. Sometimes a thyroid can become underactive because of the various treatments for an overactive thyroid. This can be a permanent condition depending on what the treatment was. Some medications like lithium can contribute to the thyroid becoming underactive. Other conditions like a pituitary disorder or even pregnancy can lead to an underactive thyroid. If the condition is left undiagnosed or untreated during pregnancy, the mother may have a miscarriage, develop preeclampsia, or give birth prematurely.

Some symptoms of an underactive thyroid are weight gain, constipation, depression, dry skin, thinning hair, hoarse voice, puffy face, increased sensitivity to cold, heavy, or irregular menstrual periods, body-wide pain or stiffness, swelling of joints, and muscle weakness. Similar to an overactive thyroid, if left untreated an underactive thyroid may lead to a goiter (enlarged thyroid), heart problems, deepening depression, infertility, higher risk of birth defects or intellectual or developmental problems of babies, and myxedema (a rare life-threatening condition that starts with drowsiness and ends with coma and perhaps death).

As you can see, it is important to make sure that the thyroid is functioning optimally. You need to have your thyroid levels at an optimal level to feel good. Conventional doctors will prescribe thyroid hormones, usually synthetic, that replace the T4. Functional doctors may prescribe either the synthetic form or a more natural form that provides T3 as well as T4. I personally was on synthetic Synthroid for many years but never quite felt optimal until switching to Armour thyroid. That's because my body seems to function better with having both T3 and T4. But that is not necessarily the case for everyone. A vegan will probably choose the synthetic route because the natural form is derived from animals. No matter what form your doctor has you on, be certain to take them on an empty stomach. That is because certain supplements or nutrients like calcium or iron will affect the absorption of the thyroid medication.

THE FUNCTIONAL MEDICINE APPROACH

Practitioners of functional medicine don't just stop with replacing the thyroid hormones with medication or, in the case of an overactive thyroid, use anti-thyroid medications. They will look for a root cause. Conventional medicine believes that being on thyroid medication will be lifelong for the individual. However, many, many patients of functional medicine have put their thyroid condition into remission, particularly if it is autoimmune-related in nature. Below, I have links to articles from a pharmacist who was able to totally put her Hashimoto's into remission by finding the root cause and treating it accordingly. This won't be the case with everyone. Some, like me, have been on thyroid medication for decades. No matter how much I do to reverse my condition, my thyroid still needs medication; yet my autoimmune levels have been dramatically lowered to close to normal levels. In my eyes, that's a win-win because my whole well-being and health have vastly improved.

So, what are some things that doctors of functional medicine look at? First and foremost, they will look at antibody levels to determine if the thyroid condition is autoimmune-related. That is because one of the primary reasons for hypothyroidism is Hashimoto's. Thyroid antibody tests, thyroid peroxidase antibody (TPO), and thyroglobulin antibody (TGAb) will be some of the blood tests they do to determine if the thyroid condition is autoimmune related. If the antibodies are elevated, that means the body views the thyroid as a foreign object and the immune system attacks it. In fact, these antibody levels can show up even if your other thyroid levels appear normal. This is why it's very important for these antibody tests to be done early on, allowing you to take steps to prevent further damage to the thyroid and lower the autoimmune reaction of your body. This will also help to prevent other autoimmune conditions. Typically, when when one person has one auto-immune condition, they tend to develop one or two more. I myself have two: Hashimoto's and celiac disease. If only I knew back then what I know now!

A note about testing: please don't take biotin for a few days before testing because it will alter the results. Not the actual hormone levels in your body, but the results that the testing shows. This happened to me not so long ago. I had started taking biotin to increase my hair growth because I had lost a very large amount of hair from having COVID-19. Biotin was working for my hair growth but my thyroid levels came back showing that my thyroid was too hyperactive. I knew that wasn't right because, other than hair loss, I had absolutely no other symptoms of hyperthyroidism. Neither I nor my doctor caught on until I accidentally learned that biotin can cause false testing results for thyroid hormones. My doctor had lowered my medication dose, which resulted in four months of dealing with an underactive thyroid. This led to low energy, not being able to get warm, increased pain, and (ugh!) weight gain! Now I stop taking biotin about a week before testing. It's recommended to stop a few days before testing but I am overly cautious and want to make sure I'm on the safe side—ha-ha!

Here are the thyroid lab tests and the optimal levels that a practitioner of functional medicine will look for versus levels conventionally considered "normal." (The optimal functional levels are based on two different lab models.)

	Optimal levels	Conventional levels (LabCorp)
Thyroid Stimulating Hormone (TSH):	1-2 IU/mL	0.4-4.5
Free T4:	15-23 pmol/L or 1.16-1.787ng/dL	0.82-1.77 ng/dL
Free T3:	5-7 pmol/L or 3.26pg/mL-4.56 pg/mL	2.0-4.4 pg/mL
Reverse T3:	11-18 ng/dL	9.2-24.1 ng/dL
TPO:	<10 IU/mL	0-34 IU/mL
TGAb:		0-0.9 IU/mL

After establishing whether the thyroid condition is autoimmune or not, other questions arise: "If it is autoimmune, why is that so? What is causing the body to attack itself?" "If the thyroid is not autoimmune, then why is it not acting properly?" Interestingly, some of the root causes may be the same and doctors will do some of the same tests. Listed next are many of the extra factors and tests that doctors of functional medicine will look at:

- Gluten intolerance, celiac, or allergy to gluten could be to blame. Gluten sensitivity and Hashimoto's seem to be closely linked. That's because gluten contains a protein, gliadin, that resembles cells in the thyroid gland. If your body is viewing gluten as a poison and attacks it, then your body may also see your thyroid as the same and attack it too.

- Other food allergies or sensitivities can play a role by causing body-wide inflammation. (See chapters 2 and 12.)

- Environmental toxins also play a role in poor thyroid function. Mercury and other heavy metals, fluoride, chlorinated water, and pesticides have been linked to thyroid problems. Some damage the thyroid tissue while others interfere with thyroid hormone production or conversion, and there are toxins that may reduce the availability of the thyroid receptors.

- Chronic stress can affect the whole endocrine system, which can contribute to thyroid disease. Doctors may do hormone tests related to the adrenal glands.

- Nutrient deficiencies can lead to a thyroid becoming under-active. Nutrients like zinc, selenium, and iodine are needed for the thyroid to perform optimally. However, many practitioners are seeing that supplementing with iodine may make an autoimmune attack worse unless selenium is given with it. That would be something to speak to your healthcare provider about. Seafood and iodized salt are a good source of iodine to consider as well as Brazil nuts for selenium.

- Goitrogenic foods are thought to cause swelling of the thyroid, called a goiter, in some people who may consume too much of them. Examples are broccoli, cauliflower, kale, spinach, cabbage, and strawberries.

- Infections that seem to have a link with Hashimoto's, like h-pylori for instance, will be looked into and treated.

Targeted treatments will be based on your own individual needs and test outcomes. Here is a list of some of the things you may be able to implement on your own or with the help of a healthcare provider:

- Remove gluten first and foremost as well as processed soy products as they can interfere with thyroid function. Remove any other foods you react to or that are inflammatory. (See chapter 2 for help in this area.)

- Replace any nutrients that may be lacking—zinc and selenium in particular. Omega 3s and vitamins A and D are good choices as well. (More about this in chapters 10 and 11 on supplements.)

- Eat a diet geared toward clean, whole foods. Consider eating seafood, salmon, and sardines that are full of iodine and omega-3 fatty acids. For selenium, eat Brazil nuts. (Chapter 2 and the "Food" portion of chapter 3 are great for learning what more about whole clean foods.)

- Eat less goitrogenic foods and prepare them by steaming and boiling them to lower the levels of the goitrogenic properties.

- Remove any toxins in your environment you have control over. (See my section on environmental toxins in chapter 3.)

- Your doctor may give you further recommendations on how to detoxify your body in a safe, gentle manner.

- Thyroid replacement hormones will most likely be a course of treatment that your doctor will need to take. I know many of you are trying to do all that you can to avoid taking any medication, but in order for your thyroid to heal and for your body to work optimally, you will need to have the proper levels of thyroid hormones in your system.

- Try to adopt healthy lifestyle habits other than the ones I have already mentioned, such as practicing good sleep habits, getting regular exercise or movement, as well as engaging in stress reduction when possible and stress management (chapters 4, 5, and 6.)

Thyroid problems cause suffering for millions; often they're undertreated, and very often they go undiagnosed. Hopefully, this chapter has helped you become more informed and better equipped to talk with your healthcare provider about it. If your doctor won't work with you then there are others who will. You deserve to have your thyroid treated properly so that it can perform at its best and you can live a good quality life.

Here are some useful articles on thyroid issues:

https://chriskresser.com/hyperthyroidism-causes-symptoms-and-treatment/

https://thyroidpharmacist.com/articles/functional-medicine-approach-to-the-thyroid/

https://chriskresser.com/most-common-hypothyroidism-causes/

https://drhyman.com/blog/2015/06/10/a-comprehensive-6-step-strategy-to-heal-your-thyroid/

CHAPTER 18

TYPE-2 DIABETES

— ❧ —

I f there is one thing that politics, science, and the medical profession agreed on during the recent COVID-19 pandemic it's that those who have type-2 diabetes are at a much higher risk of a poor outcome. How many deaths could have been prevented if there wasn't a diabetic epidemic in many parts of the world? No one knows that answer for sure, but many scientific studies indicate there would have been far fewer. This is why I've chosen type-2 diabetes as one of the chronic illnesses to write about. By focusing on lifestyle changes and other controllable factors, diabetes can be prevented and reversed if it hasn't progressed too far. That statement might not sit well with those who feel it's genetic. We will discuss genetics further in this chapter, but for now, let's dive into type-2 diabetes, starting with comparing the differing approaches taken by conventional medicine and functional medicine.

Conventional medicine and functional medicine both have a dietary approach, but it's different in each case. Conventional medicine is focused on managing blood sugar levels with carb and protein intake at the outset and eventually leading to medication if dietary means no longer work alone. When I think of conventional medicine, I think of my mom and her type-2 diabetes. My mom was diagnosed when I was a teenager. I honestly don't remember her focusing on her diet as an initial treatment plan. In fact, what I do remember her eating was a slice of Wonder Bread with margarine and sugar spread on top! My early memories of her having diabetes are when I was about seventeen and I was in nursing school. She had just started taking insulin, and I can remember her being afraid of poking herself initially, so guess who was giving her the insulin? Yep! Me, the nurse in training! The first time I gave her that shot, I was probably more scared than she was! But out of love and concern for my mom, I did it. Eventually, she got up the nerve and started giving herself the insulin. She was on insulin for the rest of her life. After studying functional medicine, I often wonder where my mom would have been without conventional medicine. Modern medicine is a wonderful tool and has saved millions of lives.

That said, science has come a long way and there are options within conventional medicine as well as functional medicine that weren't there during my mom's lifetime. Nowadays, an individual with severe type-1 or type-2 diabetes doesn't have to prick their fingers multiple times daily to test for blood sugar levels. Nor do they have to give themselves daily shots of insulin. There are devices that are attached to the body that read blood sugar levels as well as dispense insulin as needed. My sweet little niece was diagnosed with type-1 diabetes when she was just five years old. What a wonderful tool for her and her family to have! Once she was stable, she didn't have to suffer daily finger pricks and shots. Whether in the middle of the night or if she's at school, her device notifies my sister on her phone if my niece's blood sugar dips too low. Wouldn't you say that conventional medicine, although imperfect in many ways, gives us much to be thankful for?

I'm not going to include type-1 diabetes in this discussion though because it is *not* reversible and it does not have the same root causes for the most part as type-2 diabetes. Type-2 diabetes, on the other hand, may be prevented or reversed if caught early enough, and this is where functional medicine comes in. Functional medicine gives you an option and allows you to take ownership of your type-2 diabetes if that is a route that you chose to take. So let's dive into the approach of functional medicine.

I'm not going to write a lot about what type-2 diabetes is. Chances are that if you or a family member has it, then you know plenty. If you want to know more check out some of the links I have inserted in this chapter. I do want to discuss some of the myths that surround type 2-diabetes, though. The first myth is that dietary fats are a cause of type-2 diabetes, which had been the source of much debate through the years by experts. Could it be because many with this illness are obese so they think that dietary fat contributes to obesity? This is not the case, as it has been proven that dietary fats are *not* the cause of type-2 diabetes. As you learned earlier, we need healthy fats for optimal functioning. Unhealthy fats can lead to inflammation and that can be a contributing factor, but it certainly isn't a primary cause. We will discuss this further in this chapter.

The other myth: have you heard the term "diabesity?" The term came about because doctors and researchers used to think type-2 diabetes was caused by being obese. Today, they know that's not true. In fact, my mom was a very petite woman in her mid-forties, and she was not overweight when she was diagnosed. It was only in the last ten years of her life, when she was in her seventies, that she became significantly overweight.

The roots of type-2 diabetes can be complex because multiple factors are involved, such as diet, lifestyle, and genetics. You may remember earlier in this book where I mentioned epigenetics. Epigenetics shows that just because we have the genes for a particular illness doesn't mean we are destined to develop that illness. What researchers are finding is that it takes triggers for our genes to express that outcome. So for type-2 diabetes, diet and lifestyle factors can make a difference in whether they develop the condition or not.

You might ask, "Why prevent diabetes in the first place? I can enjoy my food and just take medicine or insulin to make up for it." That's a true and fair statement and may be fine for many people; however, consider what you want your life to be like down the road. What quality of life do you want? Do you want to function at your best and live the best life possible? These are questions that only you can answer. With that in mind, consider some complications of diabetes according to Mayoclinic.org: cardiovascular disease, neuropathy (nerve damage especially in the legs), nephropathy (kidney damage), retinopathy (eye damage), potential amputation of foot or toe because of lack of blood flow and nerve damage to the lower limbs, increased problems with the skin (including infections), hearing impairment, Alzheimer's, and depression.

I think of my mom often and the quality of life she could have had in her last few decades. She suffered from neuropathy in her legs, causing her much pain. So much so that about eight years before she died she was put on a medication to control that pain. The side effect of that medication led to significant weight gain, which in turn her heart couldn't handle as she already had cardiovascular disease. Eventually, she died way before she should have from congestive heart failure. Would she have made different choices if she had been more knowledgeable about health earlier in her life? Maybe, but not likely. When she was dying, did she look back with any regrets? Even though she didn't know about dietary factors or other lifestyle factors, she did have regrets, for she had also been a smoker up until about twelve years before she died, and I remember her saying she wished that she would have quit sooner. In fact, I remember her encouraging my son to quit when he was smoking. Good thing he eventually listened because he hated to see his grandma suffer so much. The point is that lifestyle choices do make a difference. Maybe not right away, but eventually they will catch up.

Eventually, science catches up too! Let's discuss some of these dietary and lifestyle factors that science is now proving to be a factor.

DIETARY FACTORS

The functional medicine approach for diet is different than that represented by conventional dietary guidelines. Much research is showing that the conventional guidelines that call for a higher carbohydrate diet may only be making type-2 diabetes worse and that low-carbohydrate diets, like the paleo or ketogenic diet models, are superior for treating the condition. Chris Kresser, M.S., L.Ac., a well-known functional medicine practitioner and teacher, states in the article that I've included below, "I have found that those with blood sugar regulation problems benefit from limiting carb intake to 10 to 15 percent of total calories." Not only is carb quantity important but carb quality, such as carbs from fruits and vegetable rather than baked goods, is important. This is because carb quality also plays an important role in regulating blood sugar levels. You can improve type-2 diabetes outcomes by eating more produce and healthy proteins while avoiding refined carbs such as baked goods and pastas. And this will come as no surprise if you've read my other chapters: avoiding gluten has shown to be beneficial in type-2 diabetes outcomes and treatment. Chris goes in depth with the functional medicine approach to type-2 diabetes in the article that I've included a link to at the end of this chapter. He talks about nutrients and gut health as well. I highly recommend you take a look.

LIFESTYLE FACTORS

Lifestyle factors play a role as well, as you will see in Chris's article. If you've read my whole book, this list shouldn't be a surprise. Regarding lifestyle in relation to type-2 diabetes intervention, a study posted in the *Lancet* says,

> *Our findings show that the intensive lifestyle intervention led to significant weight loss at twelve months and was associated with diabetes remission in over 60 percent of participants and normoglycaemia in over 30 percent of participants. The provision of this lifestyle intervention could allow a large proportion of young individuals with early diabetes to achieve improvements in key cardiometabolic outcomes, with potential long-term benefits for health and well-being.*

By now, I'm sure you see a pattern of how poor lifestyle choices in our modern-day society leads to poor outcomes. Below, I've listed specific lifestyle risk factors for type-2 diabetes that are backed by a growing amount of research. Each risk factor has a chapter of its own in this book that you can refer to for further guidance.

- Being sedentary (Safe Movement, chapter 6)
- Lack of sleep (Sleep, chapter 5)
- Poor stress management (Stress, chapter 4)
- Environmental toxins (Environmental Toxins, chapter 3)

As you can see, type-2 diabetes can largely be prevented or put into remission in the early stages. And even if you have had diabetes for a number of years, by adopting a functional medicine approach to diet and lifestyle, you can achieve better management of your diabetes. I hope this chapter on type-2 diabetes has been useful to you in your health journey! Please check out these articles I've included to help you on your journey.

https://chriskresser.com/functional-medicine-and-diabetes-how-to-treat-the-root-cause/

https://www.ifm.org/news-insights/cardio-using-functional-medicine-reverse-type-ii-diabetes/

https://www.thelancet.com/journals/landia/article/PIIS2213-8587(20)30117-0/fulltext

CHAPTER 19
BOOK SUMMARY

————————— ❧ —————————

I really hope you come away from this book with more knowledge and insight to empower you to take control of your health and wellness.

In this book you have learned about functional medicine and its scientific approach to health and wellness. We've talked about a few chronic conditions and the role that functional medicine can play in improving them. If you have a specific health condition and want to know how functional medicine can help you, do an internet search by typing in your condition or illness and then the words "functional medicine." In this way, you can continue to learn about the options that are unique to you.

I also touched on supplements and gave you some important things to consider when making a decision on whether to use them on your journey and where and what to look for when choosing a good quality supplement.

And then, most importantly, I've given you seven pillars to wellness that you can use in a manner that is unique to you. You also have the option to purchase the companion downloadable workbook on my website, www.functionalhealthbasics.com. I am confident you will feel less stress after thinking deeply about the path you want to take on your journey to better health and wellness. You can do it!

ABOUT THE AUTHOR

Cindy Cotsiopoulos is a Certified Functional Health Coach and has been in the medical field since 1984 and became a nurse in 1987. Starting in the mid-nineties, she struggled with low energy, pain, and a host of other symptoms for decades. Doctors gave her diagnoses like fibromyalgia, chronic fatigue syndrome, Hashimoto's, and celiac disease. Because of her nursing education and knowledge of anatomy and physiology she knew the body was designed to function optimally so she was always searching for the why. Why was her body not functioning optimally? Why was her son having multiple chronic health problems from birth? It wasn't until 2015 that she started to learn about functional medicine, and one by one those why's started to get answers. As she started to apply functional medicine and make changes in her lifestyle, she began to function optimally. Because of this, she wanted to find ways of educating others in an easy-to-understand, stress-free way. That is how this book and her downloadable workbook came to be.

DISCLAIMER

The information provided in this publication is for educational and informational purposes only and solely as a self-help tool for your own use. I am not providing healthcare, medical services, psychological services, or nutritional therapy services, or attempting to diagnose, treat, prevent, or cure any physical, mental, or emotional issue, disease, or condition through the information provided herein. The information provided herein pertaining to health or wellness, exercise, relationships, business/career choices, finances, or any other aspect of life is not intended to be a substitute for the professional medical advice, diagnosis, or treatment, provided by your own medical practitioner or mental health practitioner. Always seek the advice of your own medical practitioner or mental health practitioner regarding any questions or concerns you have about your specific health or any medications, herbs, or supplements you are currently taking and before implementing any recommendations or suggestions herein. Do not disregard medical advice or delay seeking medical advice because of information you have read here or anywhere else. Do not start or stop taking any medications without speaking to your own medical practitioner or mental health practitioner. If you have or suspect that you have a medical or mental health problem, contact your own medical practitioner or mental health practitioner promptly. The information contained herein has not been evaluated by the Food and Drug Administration.

The information contained herein is not intended to be a substitute for legal or financial advice that can be provided by your own attorney, accountant, and/or financial advisor.

References or links contained herein to the information, opinions, advice, programs, products, or services of any other individual, business, or entity does not constitute my formal endorsement. I am merely sharing information for your own self-help only.

www.ingramcontent.com/pod-product-compliance
Lightning Source LLC
Chambersburg PA
CBHW060231030426
42335CB00014B/1399